Planting a Seed

3 simple steps to sustainable living

PLANTING A SEED

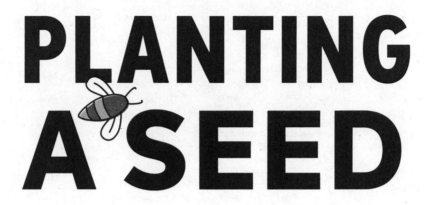

KATE GAERTNER

PAGE TWO

Some names and identifying details have been changed
to protect the privacy of individuals.

Cataloguing in publication information is
available from Library and Archives Canada.
ISBN 978-1-77458-048-6 (paperback)
ISBN 978-1-77458-049-3 (ebook)

Page Two
pagetwo.com

Edited by Amanda Lewis
Copyedited by Jenny Govier
Proofread by Alison Strobel
Cover and interior design by Taysia Louie
Cover and interior illustrations by Amy Hall-Bailey
Printed and bound in Canada by Friesens
Distributed in Canada by Raincoast Books
Distributed in the US and internationally by Macmillan

21 22 23 24 25   5 4 3 2 1

kategaertner.com

To my dearest ones, Patraic, Maddie,
and Quinn: you are my big loves.

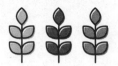

Contents

A Note from the Author

I REWROTE, REVISED, and finalized this book during the global COVID-19 pandemic. At this writing, in the US, we are still in the grip of COVID-19's chaos. The virus is present in our daily lives, albeit less so now that vaccines have been approved and are being administered in increasing numbers.

I want to acknowledge the toll the pandemic has had on each of our lives, and particularly how burdensome the impacts have been on women and people of color, psychically and financially. The pandemic induced weariness. It placed lopsided demands on us. And yet, we persisted. As parents, kids, sisters and brothers, employees and employers, we endured.

The pandemic harmed and humbled us but also shone a light on the many silver linings that can come from slowing down (for a period): living more intimately and in the moment; communing with family; going back to the basics of home-cooked meals and simpler routines; considering a broader community than our immediate family. May this book find you safe, well, healthy, and productive.

Yours in sustainability,
KATE

May 2021
Portland, Oregon

For the unlimited, unstoppable ones. The dreamers and doers… This is for you. And you. And you. This is for us.

KWAME ALEXANDER AND KADIR NELSON, *The Undefeated*

Introduction

I N T H E bathroom I share with my husband is a clear Plexiglas box with a sectional tray that allows me to store three different items for quick retrieval: Q-tips, cotton face swabs, and tampons. Lately, I'd found myself staring at the box, wondering what to do about those tampons. I hadn't opened the box to retrieve a single organic OB for over a year. I hadn't needed one since late 2019. I was officially post-menopausal.

I wondered about my daughter, aged eleven. Should I save them for her? I thought better of that idea. Who knew when she'd hit puberty or how long the tampons would last? Donating them crossed my mind. A box of tampons for many in the US, including university students, low-income women, and transgender and nonbinary individuals, is often a luxury proposition thanks to unenlightened state laws across much of the country. However, donations of a whole host of recyclable goods were curbed substantially over the last year and change.

Finally I took action, of a sustainable sort.

I took two boxes' worth (yikes! some eighty in total) of single-plastic-wrapped OBs and trotted downstairs to my kitchen. Feeling a bit sheepish for over-buying something for which I'd had an obvious waning need, I settled in by my compost bin and began unwrapping each tampon. Freed of its plastic, the tampon itself—bleached cotton and string—could successfully meet its end in a heap of foodstuff to biodegrade into productive soil.

My decision-making went as follows:

I can't just throw these tampons away as is.

What's the best way to minimize this product's impact on the earth?

What parts of this product can be recycled, reused, or composted?

When you begin your personal sustainability journey, these questions don't come easily. There's a lot of rethinking and active decision-making in remembering and then deciding how materials can best be used, disassembled, and recycled. Initially, one's sustainability journey is crowded with loud, conscious thought. Over time, those internal decision-making functions become faster and more refined. We think less and act more. Deliberations turn to routine. Sustainable practices become second-nature habits. And we become sustainably minded in intent and action.

My tampon story? I came to it after years of sustainable living and working as a corporate social responsibility professional, socializing sustainability ideas, helping to implement sustainable measures, and proudly shepherding companies on their own business circularity journeys.

I'm in the business of planting (sustainability) seeds. I do it with companies, my family and friends, and even with people I barely know. It's a yogic idea: you plant a seed for a spark of enlightenment to grow over time.

Through making shifts in how we perform tasks, to adopting actions that are more sustainable, paired with conscious changes in how we consume, our small acts add up to big, meaningful change. By prescribing three simple steps, this book brings you on a personal journey toward a simple, sustainable lifestyle.

In Part I, you will plant the seeds of change. Chapter 1 reminds you that sustainability is an old idea that remains relevant today. Chapter 2 begins to till the ground by determining what you value so you can match your personal values to the sustainable actions you want to pursue. Chapter 3 discusses the need to commit to change, and Chapter 4 discusses how to think about your personal carbon footprint. Part I wraps up with a reminder that although you are one person, you are connected to much bigger systems of production, consumption, and community, so your actions matter.

Part II focuses on nourishing the seeds we've planted. In Chapter 6 I introduce the seven impact categories where we can make change in our everyday lives. Chapters 7 through 13 are part manifesto, part action plan, providing sustainability suggestions for each of the seven impact categories: transportation, energy, home and property, food, material goods, water, and trash. Have you wondered if it is more sustainable to borrow or buy? Part II concludes with Chapter 14, a thought piece on ownership. The discussion ponders the value of owning versus sharing and how to decide based on your circumstances.

In Part III, we will grow the seeds of sustainability by putting your personal priorities into action. In Chapter 15, you will begin to curate your sustainability list by connecting the impact categories with the level of sustainability measures—small, medium, or large—you're able to implement at this time for meaningful and lasting change. Chapter 16 reinforces the idea that each of us is an empowered agent of change; to think otherwise diminishes your innate capability to embrace and amplify sustainability. Finally, the conclusion provides an inspiring tale that shows how concern can build a sustainable movement, and it recognizes you as the initiator, purveyor, and leader of change: for yourself, your family, and your broader community.

I want you to implement sustainability measures in as many areas of your life as both feel right and work for you. I don't care if you don't take radical action. I'm a big believer in moderation.

It can be fun, maybe uncertain, and sometimes scary, but with more of us walking the sustainable path, you will find your *satsang*—your group of like-minded people who bring meaning and purpose to this very important endeavor.

So try. And don't be afraid to try again and again until you find those measures that feel "just right."

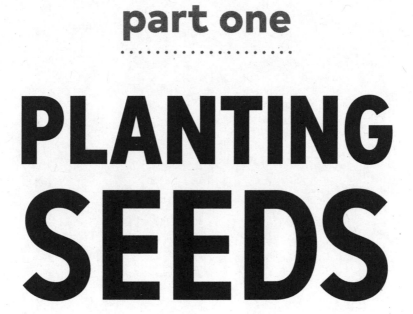

part one

PLANTING SEEDS

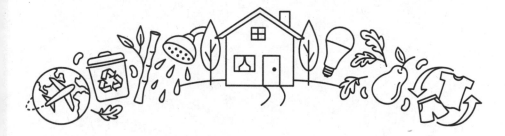

1
...

Sustainability: An Old Idea with Renewed Relevance

I am not a product of my circumstances. I am a product of my decisions.

STEPHEN COVEY

AREN'T OLD ideas some of the best? Often, they are simple remedies for what ails us. Soak in a bath of Epsom salts to wean the tiredness and soreness from muscles. "Feed a cold, starve a fever": we navigate a high body temperature with liquids and a stuffy nose with soups and starches. Upset tummy? Keep it white: eat simple carbohydrates like bread, crackers, noodles, and rice.

Most of us have grown up with maxims we heard our parents say. We've absorbed their meanings, but we may have wandered from their teachings.

"Waste not, want not." It's an admonishment as much as a lesson and can be read in different ways. One interpretation could mean: don't use too much now so you have something for later when you need it. Here's an example from my own life, despite good planning and best intentions.

During the pandemic, there were few outing options for my family. Luckily, we live just yards away from multiple entrances to Forest Park, a five-thousand-square-acre urban forest accessible from the West Hills of Portland, Oregon. When our youngest of two kids inevitably starts feeling cooped up and begins acting out, we pack up our snacks, walking gear, and water bottles and make our way to the forest for an hour-long walk. It always takes me by surprise how little legs are pained from doing the thing legs are put on this earth to do: ambulate. There is significant complaining along the way, lots of stopping for rest, and frequent requests for snack breaks. Inevitably, our kids gulp water from our Hydro Flasks despite my admonishment, "Don't drink too much. We've just gotten started. The water has to last the entire journey. Save some for everyone." Do you think my children find me wise? Nope.

Most trips into the forest, we run out of water way before hitting home, and the refrain from my kids is the same: "I'm thirsty. I need water." Yep, I hear you. Did you listen to me?

Another interpretation of "waste not, want not" is: don't waste what's useful. In classic French cooking, nothing goes to waste. The French will eat animal intestines, kidneys, livers, and tongues, and the list goes on. With a side of crusty baguette and a steamy dish of beans and flavorful sauce, unrecognizables become delicious. It is tradition in French cuisine to use the entirety of an animal, preparing the various anatomical parts to be served up in a variety of dishes that satisfy our hunger and meet our nutritional needs while honoring the animal sacrificed for our gastronomic enjoyment.

My maternal grandparents were working-class folk. They lived on a hilly plot of land in Turtle Creek, Pennsylvania. When my family used to visit them, which was at least every couple of months, my grandmother's kitchen was a cauldron of cooking, heat, and bustle. Just above where their house sat, my grandfather had planted an expansive garden on the two acres of land he owned. He grew food all year round, and those earthly treasures were harvested and prepared into ever-rotating meals each season. It was at my grandparents' house that I learned the art of canning foods, extending food harvested in the spring and summer through the winter, when fresh fruits and vegetables were hard to come by (and expensive).

I remember the glass jars, the metal lids with a separate piece in the center, and the rubber seals. I was fascinated by the wax plugs that my grandmother placed on the top of the canned food, so the fill stayed fresh and remained free of contamination. I was the designated runner in the house, the gal who was asked to run down to the storage area in the basement and grab x number of jars of this and that to be prepared and served at one of the bountiful meals my grandma always made. There was seemingly food for years down there: whole tomatoes, pickled beets, delicious fruit jams, and sliced carrots.

From a personal resilience standpoint, canning makes good sense: it's nutritious and economical. Most urban dwellers have food stocks that will last them fewer than three days in the event of an economic disruption. Here in the Pacific Northwest, everyone lives in anticipation of the Cascadia subduction earthquake that's been predicted to imminently happen... every year over the last half-century. When the event finally does happen, having a good stock of Earth's wholesome goodness locked in dozens of jars will alleviate any immediate hunger concerns (provided the jars don't break). Last year's pandemic proved that disruptions that are economic-, health-, and extreme weather–related throw our food supply into disarray.

We've moved away from axioms that espouse restraint, prize usefulness, and avoid waste to adopt new ones that amplify personal consumption. "Treat yourself," "You only live once," "You deserve it," "Why not? There's free shipping," now roll off our tongues as we scroll, click, and buy.

Here in North America, we have unlimited choices for consumption. But in the Netherlands, where my family lived for four years, the idea of limited choice is a happy societal norm. Whereas in US food stores you can find a full-length grocery row of energy bars, jams, cereals, and dried pasta, in an Amsterdam grocer, energy bars may not exist, jam and cereal options may be limited to three, and the pasta displayed may be one of each type. Brand diversity is typically limited to three or four per product category. In the fresh food section, instead of five types of oranges, just one will be displayed. Food groups and product categories are represented, but the brands and options are curated. If I still lived in Amsterdam and went to the store to buy alternative meat protein for my dinner, I would likely find one brand in three preparation forms.

Stores there act like showrooms. You go into a store to buy a crib for your baby who will be born in the coming months, and you can decide among five or six crib options but you cannot go home with a crib. You place an order for that crib that will take eight weeks to reach your house. Same for buying a mattress. You go to the mattress store and pick a model, and then wait eight weeks to receive it. The funniest (and most frustrating) experience I had living in Amsterdam was my many jaunts to the local hardware store. I'd go in because I needed garbage bags, a hammer, some picture hooks, light bulbs, a lock … everyday items. My hardware store in Amsterdam often had bare shelves where these items should be. I'd walk in, look around, ask if they carried these items. Yes, they carry them, but they are currently out of stock. A new supply will be coming in, when? Next Thursday, we think. I was flummoxed. I could never understand why these basic items weren't *always* in stock. But that's how the Netherlands rolls.

I bring up a country whose consumption practices seem old-fashioned to make a point that the ways people shop and consume goods there have an inherently sustainable quality to them. In our world, gripped by climate change and wracked by extreme weather events, old ideas ring true. Going back to basics is critical. So, a few axioms to kick us off:

Keep choices simple.

Limit over-buying.

Make things last.

For a country that was built a thousand years ago on land claimed from the Zuiderzee (North Sea), the Dutch know how to secure, endure, and thrive under challenging circumstances. From Europe and other regions around the world, we can learn different approaches to living and adopt those that make practical sense and are fundamentally self-sustaining. I want to talk about three ideas in particular.

"Make Do with Less" Made Way for "More Is Better"

It's a uniquely American phenomenon to make everything bigger. A small soda at the movie theater is now sixteen ounces. Remember when a small drink or cup of coffee started at six ounces, rose to eight ounces for a medium, and topped off at twelve ounces for a large? How about the supersizing of French pastries? In Paris, you walk into a boulangerie and can purchase a croissant for breakfast that fits into the palm of your hand. Here in the US, that same "butter" croissant can often be the size of your face. In Italy, you can order a yummy gelato in a cone on a warm sunny day. That refreshing treat will be one small scoop that fits perfectly into the diameter of a sugar cone. Here, a kid's-size cone from Ben & Jerry's is two oversized scoops stacked one upon the other and carefully tamped down into the cone so the weight of the ice cream doesn't tip the whole piece over.

"Bigger is better!" is the universal truth extolled across America at fast-food restaurants, movie-theater counters, and car dealerships and in our love of "big box" retailers. We happily order a Double Quarter Pounder burger at McDonald's because it's a deal and we think we need it: a burger with not just one but two quarter-pound beef patties symmetrically complemented by two slices of questionably real cheese slices. We order our movie snacks without much thought and select the large cola drink because it's "just a dollar more" than the standard size, a mere twenty-six ounces of sugary soda to wash down our candy and imitation-buttered popcorn.

In Europe there are no multiple-sized sandwich options to purchase. Here, Subway, the national submarine sandwich maker, offers customers three sandwich sizes to accommodate how hungry we feel we are. That trend has expanded across all manner and type of food chains.

We are a country of oversized and over-the-top. Take America's consumer truck "invention": the Hummer. This tank turned expensive SUV was a 1990s postwar darling among the rich and wanting to be seen. The military vehicle, the Humvee, was created to protect its contents—soldiers—during wartime. It was an effective machine: heavily reinforced and nearly indestructible, if not very efficient. The consumer iteration was likely to see nothing more dangerous than traffic jams around congested US cities. Even though the Hummer averaged less than ten miles per gallon, a horrendous energy efficiency metric, people bought the vehicle in droves.

Shopping at a Sam's Club or Costco is a uniquely American phenomenon. It is at once enticing, intoxicating, and utterly effective in swaying consumer behavior into the realm of the unreal: to have individuals buy groceries and basic home goods in bulk—three, five, and even ten times more than the amount required—to save a few dollars. Here's the kicker, though. This buy-in-bulk mentality tends to have two divergent paths. Either bulk goods purchased, like fresh foodstuff, go bad before they are consumed, or there is a slow (or quick) slide into a mentality of abundance where we justify using more than we need because we have so much taking up space and needing to be used and we spent less on the items than the value we arguably assign to them.

The Jevons Paradox comes to mind here. William Stanley Jevons was an English economist during the Industrial Revolution around the mid- to late nineteenth century. He observed that with increases in coal efficiency, which was the standard fuel of the day, instead of there being a reduction in use, more coal was being consumed. Hence, the paradox: as efficiencies are made in a resource, the unintended consequence is consumption of that resource increases. The Jevons Paradox can be applied to a whole host of contrary outcomes; for example, people tend to eat more low-fat ice cream than full-fat, leading to increased weight gain. Or people who buy more stuff at a lower price tend to also consume and waste more than individuals who shop in a more measured way only "for what is needed."

We love and fully embrace our bulk discount megaretailers such as Walmart and Target. Don't buy two kiwis, buy this package of sixteen. Need some lip balm? Don't buy one, buy six with this pack. At the retail counter where sales are rung up, the sales assistant will proffer, "You want another? You'll save twenty percent!" Usually, I reflexively say, "No, thank you." I don't like to buy in bulk, except when it comes to vegetable stock and tomato sauce. You can never have too much of either. But the constant prompt makes me do the math: I'm not saving; I'm spending more money. And for what purpose? Do I need double the hand sanitizer I thought I needed? Do I really need a second pair of fuzzy slipper socks?

Capitalism teaches us that more benefits us, as well as society as a whole. It's a growth mentality run amok.

In our lives, we sometimes go through big, scary systemic shocks that compel us to rethink how we act and consume. The Great Depression lasted ten long years in the US. Both my mom and dad were Depression-era babies, having been born in 1937 and 1939, respectively. I've read about how tough that time was. Out-of-work men and boys riding trains across the country, women waiting in bread lines for food to sustain their families, farmers abandoning their fields because the proceeds of harvesting weren't worth the effort.[1] My mother's grandfather lost his fortune in the stock market crash of 1929. He was a devastated man.

I remember how my father's parents would keep every pack of sugar, salt, and pepper; pocket every extra ketchup sachet; and gather in a paper napkin individually wrapped butter packets when we ate in a restaurant together. My brothers and sister and I would snicker about how they silently pirated away these small gems of food. We didn't understand why, until we saw where all that "booty" went: their home kitchen. Mum-mum, my grandmother, once opened her freezer in front of me, and there were mounds of individually wrapped little butter pats in there, just waiting to be eaten at some later date ... or never. Yes, she hoarded butter long after the Depression ended and life became comfortable. Waste not, want not.

During World War II, Americans were asked to make all kinds of personal sacrifices in support of the collective good. The war effort required commandeering manufacturing plants to ensure that war goods were in sufficient supply for the soldiers who were fighting on the front lines. The government rationed all kinds of consumer goods—meat, sugar, firewood, and medicine—asking people to make do with less. People were asked not to drive during the war, and "pleasure drives in the countryside were more or less outlawed." [2] Gas that ran cars was redistributed to the war effort. So, too, the rubber of car tires, which was repurposed to insulate all types of war machines. Americans sacrificed. There were grumblings, but all in all, individuals understood the need for the rationing. We can make do with less and be well.

More recently, we lived through the twin global health and economic shocks of the COVID-19 pandemic. Remember those first days and weeks, when bread, milk, tissue paper, paper towels, toilet paper, wet wipes, and hand sanitizer were out of stock on most grocery shelves or, if they were in stock, rationed to just one or two items per person? The message was: don't buy more than you need; spread the love; leave stock for others. As the year progressed and we found ourselves at home, quarantined or in rolling lockdowns, working virtually and juggling all the elements of our lives from inside our houses, we began to consume differently.

> We cooked and ate at home more often.
> We planted gardens with our favorite food items.
> We bought fewer clothes.
> We purchased less makeup.
> We stopped buying jewelry.
> We made do with a messier hairdo.
> We groomed less because we went out less.
> We stopped driving our cars.

Of course, we had upticks in other types of purchases:

- Face masks
- Take-out food
- New electronics to be productive at home
- Video-streaming services for entertainment to escape with
- Booze (well, at least for the non-teetotalers among us!)

The arrival of COVID-19 forced us to live life differently. Yes, it was often painful to be forced to change so much so quickly. But unanticipated silver linings revealed themselves among the chaos and uncertainty:

- I saw my husband all day, every day.

- My family took almost daily impromptu walks in the forest together.

- My husband shared home and family responsibilities with me.

- I bonded with my pre-teen daughter. We lunched together daily and took afternoon strolls through the neighborhood.

- I worried less about how I looked. Listen, I'm still vain, but I went from coloring my hair every eight weeks to quarterly, and wearing far less makeup and minimal jewelry.

Here's the short of it. Doing less and having less does not have to equate with being worse off. It does not have to equal sacrifice. Less can be better. A few things can be enriching. We may have to force ourselves to experience those happy unintended consequences of trying a different way of being.

A sustainable life is a new way of living in this world. For you, it may initially carry the mental moniker of sacrifice, doing without, less-than, hardship, not fun. But sustainability is none of those things. It is a marriage of what you value with what is valuable for sustaining the world you know and love. It is a life well lived and imbued with meaning. It is taking a light touch that is the right combination of satisfying your needs while considering the needs of a collective community.

"Made to Last" Made Way for "Made to Be Replaced"

How many times have you bought a hair dryer thinking you'd have it forever, only to find two years later that it has mysteriously stopped working? It usually has something to do with hair getting trapped in some chamber and a burning smell. Or, a buildup of lint in the mesh on the backside of the nozzle. Who knows. I'm surprised, because hair dryers are simple machines. You'd think they could handle a little hair and lint.

Here's another example I think most of us can appreciate: your home printer (if you even have one!). My printer is of the ink-jet variety from HP. On average, my home printer lasts about one and a half to two years, maximum. Something always breaks, and every troubleshooting guide fails. Or the manufacturer stops supporting the software for their particular model after a certain period, rendering it useless. Ca-ching! Go purchase another.

The same goes for my relatively "old" iPads. We own two, both under five years old. Problem is, they are bumping up against that inevitable date when their operating systems won't be supported by Apple. Our last iPad, now more than eight years old, was one of the "walking dead" electronics. At some point in the last two years, we were afraid of updating its operating system because we knew that when we did, we'd lose the use of the device. Crazy, right? The operating system was made obsolete by the company that made it.

We've moved at hyper-speed from "made to last" to "made to be replaced." Materials can't be repaired because their blend is shoddy—not repairable—by their very nature. Electronics manufactured and bought by individuals are designed to be "retired" within a certain number of years, the shorter the better. Planned obsolescence is a deliberate demand strategy employed by product manufacturers. Companies don't support their brilliant electronic creations because they don't want to support you not buying another brand-new machine to replace the old. The jig is up: newer is better; old is out.

"Multi-Use" Made Way for "Single-Use"

Goodness, I used to love my Ziploc bags. With little kids in my life, plastic sandwich, freezer storage, and snack bags were like my cool little kitchen treats. There's a size for everything, and every bag has a unique function. They zip. They lock. They double lock. I mean, the product extensions on these plastic babies are endless!

How about the boon in single-serving packaging of food items? We have "snack pack" single-serving sizes for everything: cookies, crackers, peanut butter, instant noodle soup, Lunchables, nuts, dried fruits. And the killer of all these options is that they are wrapped, bathed, secured, packaged, and ensconced in plastic. The "promise" of plastic's coming ubiquity is alluded to in one famous scene from *The Graduate*, a movie set in the 1960s, when Benjamin (Dustin Hoffman) is pulled aside by Mr. McGuire (Walter Brooke), a friend of his father's, to learn about the future of plastic.

Mr. McGuire: I just want to say one word to you. Just one word.
Benjamin: Yes, sir.
Mr. McGuire: Are you listening?
Benjamin: Yes, I am.
Mr. McGuire: Plastics.

The Belgium-born American Leo Baekeland invented the very first form of plastic, Bakelite, in the early 1900s. From there, the variety and types of (fossil-fuel-derived) plastics exploded, starting with the invention of Scotch tape by 3M in 1930. As companies in Europe and the US learned how to make plastic more malleable, invented injection moldings and extruders to shape melted polymers, and discovered new types of plastics such as polyethylene (PE), the use of the material became commonplace in consumer goods packaging. Ever since, plastic production and pollution have proliferated.

Before plastics, we operated in durables and valued longevity. We learned to "make do and mend," and we understood reusability equated with material usefulness. Post–World War II, we moved quickly and steadily away from durable and long-lasting to disposable and one-use in the materials we used, the products we bought, and the food we ate.

Glass, aluminum, and steel: these materials have near infinite lifespans. They can be melted and reformed into new products while retaining the qualities and attributes inherent within them. Said another way: they are highly "upcyclable" materials.

Plastic containers like Tupperware can of course be reused. But most plastics cannot be easily recycled today. When they are, most can only be "downcycled": recycled into items of lesser quality than the original products. Milk jugs are incorporated into plywood fencing; PVC pipes are recycled into shipping envelopes; water bottles are chipped to make pillow stuffing.

Today, there are two types of highly recyclable plastics: PET/PETE (labeled #1) and HDPE (labeled #2). Think plastic water bottles for #1 PET plastic; milk jugs and clothing detergent containers for #2 HDPE plastic. The "oh my goodness" moment comes when we find out that just nine percent of all #1 and #2 plastic is actually recycled in America. The rest of that highly recyclable plastic material ends up in our landfills, polluting our land and off-gassing methane that goes into our air and heats up our environment.

Guess how much of the 14 million tons of plastic produced in the US is used just once and then thrown away in the trash? Have a number in your head? Forty percent: just under half of all plastic consumed is used only once.[3]

Does it make you want to use fewer Ziploc plastic bags? It did for me. The plastic bags I use now, I reuse religiously: use, wash, dry, and repeat.

Disposability seems to be our schtick here in the US. It's a by-product of a consume-more culture that has emphasized a "buy more and faster" mentality for Americans. But if you start to look around, there are more options. Take Raz Mason, for one.

RAZ MASON

Always prepared with handy durables

RAZ MASON is a jill-of-all-trades: a chaplain, teacher, resiliency coach, and climate leader in Al Gore's Climate Reality

Project. Raz lives in The Dalles, a rural town in eastern Oregon that falls in the "rain shadow" of Mount Hood. She's lived and worked bi-coastally: in Portland, Oregon, and Seattle, Washington, as well as in Philadelphia and the DC metro area, and studied at Harvard Divinity School in Cambridge, Massachusetts. One thing Raz is: always prepared.

She and I met one evening for dinner at Andina, a favorite Peruvian restaurant of mine in Portland. As we ate, we talked about life and our respective work on climate solutions. The Peruvian cuisine is one of diversity, just like the culture and history of Peru. We both had agreed to share plates, and lots of them, so that she, having never tried the food before, could experience all it had to offer. We each ordered four plates. They were not small. Even though I usually bring my he-man appetite to nice restaurants, we were left with quite a bit of food that, if we decided not to take it home with us, would go to waste.

I don't like to doggy-bag my leftover food. I prefer to eat everything I order. But just as importantly, I didn't want to use the restaurant's disposable plastic containers and tops and a plastic bag to haul my leftovers home.

Raz asked, "Do you want to take the remaining food home?"

"Well," I said, "would you?"

Raz reached under the table and into her backpack, and she took out three glass containers. "These are for you," she said. "A gift for paying for dinner. You can use them to doggy-bag the food home." And that's Raz in a nutshell. Prepared, unfazed, and always sustainable.

When we asked our server if he would use our containers to pack up the food, a broad smile took over his face, mixed with amusement and knowingness. "Yes, and good idea," our server said. "I wish more people did just what you did right now."

Sustainability Defined

At MIT in Cambridge, Massachusetts, great minds ponder the depths and definitions of sustainability. One of those definitions that resonates with me is by John R. Ehrenfeld, the former executive director of the International Society for Industrial Ecology and author of *Flourishing: A Frank Conversation about Sustainability*. For many years, he acknowledges, understanding and defining sustainability has not been easy:

> The word "sustainability" itself is misleading. As a noun, it is meaningless in practice unless it refers to some *thing* that is to be sustained. It is, in fact, a question in need of answering: can we sustain growth? Can we sustain our population? Can we sustain our lifestyle?[4]

I like that an academic such as John seeks to make sustainability relevant to individuals and not just to nations, municipalities, and organizations. Because it is you and me who come together to organize. Human beings are the essence of those large institutions and organizational systems. We need to understand what sustainability is and how to enact it.

To be efficacious, we must absorb sustainability into our life so it is the very essence of who we are and what we stand for. We do this by aligning our values with sustainable actions and practices. We build the lifestyle we seek by making commitments to choices that reinforce our values. Through this intertwining series of choices and commitments, we become sustainable by embodying the practice of sustainability.

John defines sustainability as that which is flourishing, and measured by "quality," not quantity.

> Flourishing ... comes when one can say that life's cares are being attended to—when every human being is successfully caring for themselves, other humans, and the non-human world that is vital to our maintenance.[5]

Isn't that what we inherently seek in life, to care for and be comforted by others?

Companies are also re-embracing an old, pre-1980s way of "operating" that emphasizes a "more than profit" mentality. Consideration for an organization's stakeholders—employees, customers, the communities where businesses reside—for their health, productivity, and well-being, is gaining equal importance to profit-making. We see this movement in the growing number of companies that are registering as benefit companies in their states; becoming members of B Lab, a membership that signifies companies are resolute in helping to build a regenerative and inclusive economic system; and actively disclosing environmental, social, and governance information that is in addition to the oft-required financial disclosures companies must make. In essence, companies are looking back in time and pulling forward, and they are applying the value of mutual respect, supporting sustainable practices, and helping to build a more resilient world by reviving the social compact between organizations and individuals: mutual care for mutual benefit.

Rethinking "Today's Sensibilities"

Today is the perfect day to rethink how and what we buy. We've moved away from sustainable practices that were more typical features of earlier decades. We wandered into a wondrous forest of more-is-better, use-and-chuck, and planned obsolescence. Frankly, we lost our way.

We are trashing and torching the planet. We are creating open sewers and piles of waste that ruin the world's beauty and can jeopardize our health, as well as the health and biodiversity of other animals. We are not apart from nature; we are part of it. But we've been conditioned to consume in unhealthy, oversized ways, and we've been measuring value the wrong way: quantity over quality.

Let's value quality. Let's value sustainability. Let's get back to flourishing.

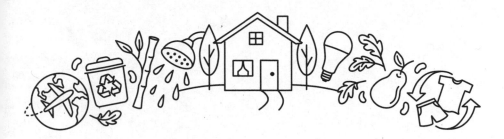

2

····

Know What You Value

Three weeks of information
I never had before have changed
forty years of ingrained driving
habits... I didn't have to change
my values. I just had to see
how my action did and did not
conform to my values.

DONELLA H. MEADOWS, *The Global Citizen*

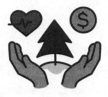

I DON'T WANT you to just read about sustainability; I want you to enact it. One of the best ways I know to do that is to link sustainable actions to what you already value. If sustainability measures reinforce what you value today, then pursuing them is like an amuse-bouche served at a fine dining restaurant: a delightful, satisfying morsel that adds to your dinner experience.

We all organize our lives around the internal values we have, whether stated or not. These are ideas, things, people, and even practices we hold dear. Below are some examples:

- I prize sleeping eight hours a night because good sleep keeps me happy and healthy.

- I read to my kids every night before bed because it instills a love of reading.

- I call my mom daily because I want her to know that I love her.

- We eat as a family nightly because it builds a strong family unit.

Of course, our value system extends beyond ourselves and our immediate family.

- I shop at farmers markets because I want to support local businesses in my community.

- I plant native trees and flowering plants on my property to support my state's local pollinators.

- I don't water my lawn in the hot summer months because it's important to conserve freshwater resources.

And like life itself, our value systems can shift and change. What we held as important in our teenage years may be different in our mid-thirties. Our values will continue to expand and refine as we move through marriage, parenting, and our advancing career. Some of our values will remain fixed throughout our life; others will be newly acquired. As we grow and learn, we take on new mantles and let others fall away.

I'd argue that sustainability is much like learning a new subject matter, whether in a formal academic setting or as a new hobby, like playing the piano or crocheting. We learn and practice but keep it simple at first. We build up our finger muscles and memorize the feeling of the hook in our hands and the knots that form a weave. We master basic ditties on the ivory keys with one hand before we add the other to support a richer melody. As we gain comfort in our crocheting ability, we progress our knowledge and challenge ourselves to move from crafting a straight scarf to a rounded hat. The progression of our learning and understanding is validated by our growing confidence and the sophistication of our capabilities.

We know more. We try more. We gain confidence. We progress our knowledge. We apply our learning in deeper, more meaningful ways.

The "test" for us is seeing the results of our efforts.

Your Sustainability Lens

If you were a photographer hired to take photos of a special occasion, how would you best capture the moment? Would you shoot in color or black and white? Would you take still shots or video? Would you capture scenes as a photojournalist would—fluid and unexpected—or more as a portraitist, formally choreographing images? Would you use a digital camera or go old-school and use an analog Nikon?

You have a gut feeling about your aesthetic preferences. You may consider a couple different approaches, but you generally know what you like and what you would prioritize.

The same goes for picking our value-driving preferences. Can you articulate which of the following drivers ring true for you? (There can be multiple that resonate.) Which one would you consider a motivating factor for taking sustainability action in your life and with your family? I have identified four value drivers:

1 Saving money
2 Living a healthy life
3 Building community
4 Supporting the biodiversity of the planet

For each, an avatar based on a real person is presented to give you a sense of how your personal values align with sustainability measures you could take.

Cost Savings

Are you driven by saving money? Perhaps a lens of frugality drives your sustainability decisions, as it does for Robin Haight.

Money matters. We can get so caught up in what are the right things to do and what needs to be done to be sustainable. We can lose ourselves in whether we "believe" in climate change and what may be causing it. And we can fight about the political stances that Republicans and Democrats have on global warming. But, when all is said and done, sustainability comes down to what is important to us: Does sustainability align with our values? Robin Haight taught me that.

Robin is a fifty-year-old middle school teacher. She's an eastern Oregonian through and through, having been born and raised in the state and, now married with three girls, living in eastern Oregon for the last quarter of a century.

People are important to her. It flows from her work with the church. Robin is both deeply religious—she was raised Christian and has a strong belief in God—and a science teacher, educating students about "little bits" of all sciences, including physical, earth, and life.

Robin is a registered Republican and votes conservative. She doesn't like politics and prefers to relate to people at the individual level. She admits to knowing about the impacts from climate change that exist today, such as sea level rise, ocean acidification, and the melting Arctic. She also feels climate change impacts that are directly affecting her local community, such as changing weather cycles, more extreme hot and cold spells, and delayed seasons. Still, she's skeptical about whether climate change is human-induced.

With their family of five headed by two public school teachers, saving money is top of mind. As Robin makes clear, many of the sustainability measures she and her husband pursue come from the perspective of wanting to drive their household costs as low as possible. And boy, are they successful at it.

In the summer months from March to October, Robin dries the family clothes and other textiles (bedsheets and rugs) on a fixed clothesline in their yard. She says it helps save them money on energy costs and supports keeping the house cool. Her house is primarily heated by a wood stove located in the basement. The house requires between two and three cords of wood per winter at a cost of $250 to $300 per cord. She and her husband make chopping wood a family outing. They buy a wood salvage permit to collect and chop wood for the winter. And the family grows a garden each year. They eat fresh all summer, preserving the bounty for the winter months and selling the rest at their local farmers market, netting the family about $30 each week, which partly offsets a weekly grocery bill that averages $125. As Robin says, "It's a hobby of my husband's [the garden], but it's super practical as well." The garden grows food and feeds her kids as well as provides a source of revenue.

For Robin, sustainability builds personal resilience. It's a mindset. She knows climate change will create problems in the future. She feels confident she and her family have developed a workaround and the ability to solution-set for the period of time that is needed to get through a disruption. She and her husband have prepped so that they could survive a couple of weeks or longer with stored food, water, and a heat source, if needed, in a natural disaster from climate change.

For Robin, being frugal is being smart. Saving money over the long run is a priority.

Cost Savings is her value driver. She is a Penny-Wiser.

Sustainability decisions that align with her value driver include these measures:

- Air seal the home.
- Insulate the attic.
- Install high-efficiency (HE) appliances.
- Use drip irrigation on the lawn.

Healthy Lifestyle

Are you motivated to live a healthier, fitter, more active life? An approach that marries a healthy, active lifestyle with sustainable actions might be your lens, as it is for Danny Metcalf.

One with nature. Danny is a high-energy, thirty-year-old former competitive triathlete who loves the outdoors and all things active that allow him to commune with nature. Danny works for a political consultancy in Washington, DC, helping to bring analytical rigor to political awareness campaigns. Prior to his political work, he worked for a global kombucha beverage company, one that was particularly dedicated to sustainable practices and giving back to environmental organizations to support forest and water conservation.

Danny is on a quiet mission to contribute meaningfully to climate change mitigation. He commutes to work via his electric bike (ebike). The twelve-mile round-trip journey is a pleasure for him. He thoroughly enjoys the fresh air and being alone with his thoughts at the beginning and end of each day.

Danny bikes because it keeps him active. Biking is made easy because his ebike is battery-propelled to help him along his journey over hills and across longer distances. His ebike makes daily commuting via bike a reality and allows him to remain physically active while working a full-time professional job. More so, Danny's satisfaction comes from knowing that the largest personal carbon emissions category—combustion-engine emissions—doesn't apply to his life.

For Danny, staying active and fit, communing with nature, and creating as little impact on the planet as possible are his personal priorities.

Healthy Living is his value driver. He is a Be-Bester.

Sustainability decisions that align with his value driver include these measures:

- Bike to work.
- Purchase only sustainably made products.
- Be a vegetarian.
- Avoid genetically modified (GMO) foods.
- Install photovoltaic (PV) solar panels on the home.

Building Community

Are you dedicated to supporting your community? Are you steadfast in making its economy vibrant by spending your dollars locally and with people and businesses you trust? If so, your sustainability lens may involve trusting in your community and building fellowship among like-minded peers, as it does for Marion Silas.

Love local. Marion Silas is a bright, curious twenty-seven-year-old who works in the mortgage industry and lives in northern Virginia. She recently purchased her first home and is passionate about fixing up the place and making it distinctly her own.

Marion is a rabid consumer of local food and personal care products. Her path to becoming a passionate advocate of the local community and economy began with a food transition in her teens.

Starting in high school and continuing into college, Marion gave up meat to become a vegetarian. That experience lasted seven years. Her catalyst was her disdain for the factory (a.k.a. industrial) farming of animals. She hated how inhumanely the animals were treated and the methods used to keep the animals healthy (enough) before they were slaughtered: the extensive use of steroids to "beef up" the cows as quickly as possible and the rampant use of antibiotics to stave off illness in the animals from their caged, fecal-wading, food-engorged days.

When she began to introduce meat into her diet again, she made a conscious decision to only buy and eat animal meat from local farms that employed sustainable practices for raising animals and treated them humanely, providing them with respect and a good life. Marion says she only wants to put "clean" meat in her body.

She researched ethical meat producers in Virginia. She would travel to the various farms to meet the local farmers and to see the conditions in which the animals lived. From her research and visits, Marion began buying meat that was pasture-raised and hormone- and antibiotic-free. It was from this primary research that she built a community of farms in Virginia that she trusts. Her research grew to sourcing products beyond meat to fruits and vegetables, local body products, and personal accessories. She gains great satisfaction from knowing her food choices provide positive health benefits.

Marion feels personally enriched by knowing the people who raise the animals and grow the food she eats. These community relationships are meaningful to her. She talks about the friendships as a forged "fellowship" with people who share her values. She places great value on supporting her local community. "I feel good knowing that what the farmers say in how they farm and raise livestock is accurate and true. I know the people. I trust them and their word."

For Marion, buying local and building community is important. Building trusted, mutually rewarding relationships with farmers and product purveyors brings her joy.

Building Community is her value driver. She is a Bridge Builder.

Sustainability decisions that align with her value driver include these measures:

- Buy local.
- Shop at farmers markets.
- Eat only seasonally grown food.

- Grow a garden and share excess vegetables and fruits with neighbors.
- Share lawn tools with neighbors.

Supporting Biodiversity

Are you concerned about biodiversity loss? Do you seek to support the health and productivity of your local environment? Maybe the promotion of biodiversity and care for Earth's natural resources could drive your sustainability decisions, as they do for Sam Crane.

Healthy land. Sam Crane is a retired public school science teacher and, during the summer months, park ranger. He lives in Granby, Colorado, located some ninety miles from Denver and just twenty miles from the western entrance to Rocky Mountain National Park. Sam knows about the environment. He grew up on a farm in Upstate New York loving to hunt, fish, hike, and ski. He holds a degree in zoology and two minors in botany and chemistry. He's worked fifty-five seasons in the national park system, mainly stationed in the Western states.

Sam is a lover of the outdoors, and he sought to instill that same love in his students. "I tried to impress upon students the importance of nature and the environment." Sustainability to Sam is a universal truth. "Don't do anything that will negatively affect the ability of future generations to utilize the resources we enjoy today."

For Sam, living sustainably means treading lightly on this earth. He recycles everything he can. He walks and bikes as much as possible. He bought his 1,300-square-foot home in order to be close to the school where he taught, so commuting by car would not be necessary. He has a lawn but has kept it turf-free. He does not actively water his property but optimizes its natural features to ensure the trees and plants that do exist thrive.

Sam refers to his lawn as "unkempt and weed-infested"; land not "scaped." He likes it that way because, as he says, "the dandelions support the local honeybees." The trees he has planted, which are all native to the region, were installed to create a natural privacy fence for his house. Because he avoids irrigation, he dug a trench filled with mulch around his tree planting, which serves as a bioswale for effectively feeding the trees with nutrients and naturally capturing rainwater.

Sam thinks in systems: environmental, sustainable, political. He knows a big part of his job with students was to arm them with knowledge in order to activate personal action. He leaves me with this: "We need to get our political system aligned with sustainable systems. Be both an informed and active citizen."

For Sam, a healthy environment is the only option we should consider. His priority is to effect high-functioning "ecosystem" services.

Supporting Biodiversity is his value driver. He is a Nature Lover.

Sustainability decisions that align with his value driver include these measures:

- Convert hardscape surfaces (cement, asphalt) to permeable pavement.
- Walk and bike to work.
- Plant native trees and bushes.
- Use no synthetic chemicals.

If you can tell me which of the four categories are personal priorities for you, I can tell you which sustainability measures you should pursue. In some sense, it's that simple. You have identified what is important to you as an individual or family. You have told me that you prioritize and execute on these values in your everyday life. Now, you can match sustainability measures to your value drivers and start taking action. As Emeril Lagasse says, "Bam!" It's that easy.

Why is it important to identify our personal value drivers before we start implementing sustainability measures? Because it's about commitment to action. Living our values helps us commit to a life in which we are flourishing.

We do the things that are important to us. We complete what we prioritize on our to-do lists. We do those things that reinforce who we believe we are.

Building a List of Sustainability Measures
· ·

OK, so you've determined your value drivers. From there, we can build a list of sustainability measures to pursue.

In the legend below, determine which trait (or traits) resonates most with your personal priorities. I've created fun sustainability monikers you can try on and wear.

Value Driver	Core Value Trait	Sustainability Moniker
Cost Savings	Frugality	The Penny-Wiser
Healthy Living	Fitness and outdoor activity	The Be-Bester
Building Community	Trust, fellowship, and symbiosis	The Bridge Builder
Supporting Biodiversity	Concern for a clean environment (air, land/soil, and water)	The Nature Lover

Let's say you've determined that saving money is your primary motivator for implementing sustainability in your life. Great! Below is a starter list of sustainability actions you—the Penny-Wiser—can choose from right now.

- Purchase an electric bike (ebike).

- Install high-efficiency (HE) appliances (such as dishwasher and clothing washer and dryer) to lower your water and energy costs.

- Install a drip irrigation system for your lawn and deck plants.

- Lease an electric vehicle (EV) and save money on fuel and car maintenance.

Why these measures? Well, because each of these sustainability tips has a definite cost savings associated with it that grows more substantial over time.

- Ebikes are affordable transportation systems that cost between $2,000 and $4,000 to buy.

- HE washers and dryers save $40 in energy and water costs each year.

- Drip irrigation systems can cut water bills in half.

- EVs cost around $10 per month to charge and require no fuel and little maintenance.

What if the key value driver you identify is supporting biodiversity and a healthy environment? A similar set of sustainability measures can be compiled for you—the Nature Lover—to pursue.

- Compost all food waste to avoid landfill buildup.

- Use only natural pesticides and fertilizers for lawn and house plant upkeep.

- Purchase clothing made from natural fibers only.

- Grow a garden with native plants that support pollinators.

Again, why these suggested measures? They reinforce cleaner air and land, support more productive soil, and reduce waste and reliance on fossil fuels.

The same kind of correlation can be made between the Healthy Living value driver and sustainability measures that support better personal health, and between the Building Community value driver and measures that feed, promote, and reinforce the people and businesses of a local economy.

Take a look at the starter list of sustainability measures to follow, grouped by the four value drivers we've identified in this chapter. (This is by no means an exhaustive list.)

Sustainability Measures by Value Driver

Penny-Wisers (Cost Savings)	Be-Besters (Healthy Living)
• Replace a gas range with electric. • Grow your own garden. • Plant drought-resistant plants in your yard.	• Eat non-animal alternative proteins. • Walk or bike to work. • Buy sustainably made clothing.
Bridge Builders (Building Community)	**Nature Lovers (Supporting Biodiversity)**
• Invest in community solar. • Become a CSA (community-supported agriculture) member of a local produce farm. • Install a rain cistern to capture stormwater runoff.	• Plant only native trees and bushes. • Avoid using any synthetic chemicals inside and outside of your home. • Use only natural fertilizers and pesticides in your garden.

I've promised you a simple three-step system for building sustainability into your life. We have checked off one of those steps: determining your value driver. The second step toward building your sustainability muscle is to learn how to categorize measures. I like to talk about them as "impact categories." Once you know what those impact categories are, you can pick and choose measures from each that you want to pursue. We will learn more about impact categories in Part II.

The last of the three steps to personal sustainability is to separate and demarcate measures into buckets of sustainability actions to be pursued. The S-M-L sustainability framework categorizes actions into small (easy to do), medium (require more effort), and large (involve financial and technological commitments). This is a scalable framework to bring order and understanding to sustainability measures that are important to you—that reinforce your personal values—and fall into your purview of capabilities. These measures are doable, they reveal a willingness for changing behaviors and processes to create new habits, and they use resources (time and financial) in a careful and repeatable manner.

The S-M-L sustainability framework is valuable in two distinct ways:

- It allows you to quickly scan and identify measures that are affordable and can be easily completed, providing you with quick wins to spur you along.

- It fosters a growth mindset by developing a roadmap—created by you, for you—that grows and deepens your commitment to sustainability measures that are more positively impactful both to the earth and to others beyond yourself and your family.

With the S-M-L sustainability framework, you determine where you are going to begin your journey and where you'd like to progress. It's the same as writing your personal and professional goals at the beginning of each new year: What do you want to achieve this year, in three years, and in ten? For each tranche of goals, we progress toward the initial targets we set for ourselves, which help us get closer to our ultimate end goals. We don't become marathon runners by entering into a local 10K run when we haven't run around the block. Running a marathon takes a ton of little goals to be set and met, which then allow us to run twenty-six-plus miles without injury or flame-out. During many months, we develop our stamina, endurance, and mental fortitude.

We want to ultimately achieve big sustainability goals, but we need smaller, more manageable goals to keep us excited to learn and do more. It's motivating to experience quick wins: sustainability tips we've employed in our life and mastered.

Before we build a customized sustainability plan, we have a few more learning stops. In the next chapter, I'll discuss what kinds of changes you must embrace to be sustainable.

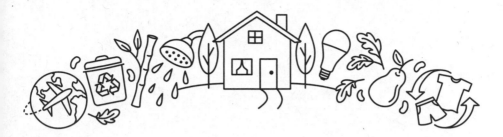

3

....

Committing to Change

The most difficult
thing is the decision
to act. The rest
is merely tenacity.

AMELIA EARHART

CHANGE SEEMS to be a scary idea for most, but it's a commonplace occurrence in our lives. Every second of every day we are vastly changing and growing. Don't believe me? Your body is creating on average 2.5 million new red blood cells every second.[1] That's a lot of change! If we're already "used to" that much change happening at a biological level, we can surely contemplate a handful of changes to build sustainability in our lives, right?

Let's talk about three types of changes in detail:

1 **Behaviors:** How one unconsciously gets a task done.
  Example: Taking a three-minute versus a fifteen-minute shower.

2 **Processes:** The approach employed for completing necessary life tasks on a daily, weekly, and monthly basis.
  Example: Commuting by public transportation or bike versus personal automobile.

3 **Financial investments:** Spending on new, more efficient technologies or innovations that afford one the ability to do more with less, use alternative non-polluting energies, or reduce usage of some material or energy.
  Example: Purchasing LED bulbs, leasing an electric vehicle, or installing photovoltaic solar panels.

Behaviors
· · · · · · · · · · ·

Behaviors refer to the ways in which we conduct ourselves. Much of them are unconsciously decided. They are unwritten rules by which we live, often inherited over our lifetimes, learned from our early days as kids and young adults. Think about how you cook and eat. Much of the comfort foods you love come from your very earliest experiences of trying them. Good memories are attached to them, like a cold night when your mom cooked that delicious chili with kidney beans, topped with shredded cheddar cheese and served with a crusty baguette. Or maybe it was that time unexpectedly, after a tough day at school, Dad made his "famous" homemade mac and cheese dish, sizzling hot out of the oven with breadcrumbs on top and the oozing gooeyness of the cheese giving each mouthful a lovely, prolonged sensation. To this day, you may still cook chili and mac and cheese exactly as you experienced them the first time. But when you are diagnosed with a digestive health issue, eating rich and fatty foods will not be beneficial to your sustained health. You must then make different and better dietary decisions that support your long-term wellness. These decisions must first be consciously made, even when you want to resist them. This is the relearning period of changing out old habits for new, more beneficial ones. Over time and with much conscious iteration of your new behaviors, new habits become embedded in your mind, so much so that you no longer have to think about them, consciously, to perform them. They become your new and standard way of doing things—your habits. That is conscious, incremental adaptation.

Processes
· · · · · · · · · · ·

Personal processes are novel ways you go about accomplishing what needs to be done to run your life smoothly on a daily, weekly, and monthly basis. You fill the car up with gas once a week. You go grocery shopping on Mondays and Thursdays. You drop off your dry cleaning every Tuesday. You pay your household bills the second of every month. You set up standards and routines to keep track of all that needs to get done on a continuous basis. You can call it a mental checklist of life's to-dos. Some of these practices you just do and don't think about much. A pair of socks gets a hole in them, so you throw them away and buy another pair. You use aluminum foil until the roll is depleted, and you put it on your shopping list to get more. You buy that gallon of laundry detergent because having more is better and more "cost effective."

When you're open to new practices, you are open to trying new brands, new concepts, and new ways of accomplishing a task. For instance, many of us now use ebanking services. Adopting this system helps us build a new practice, one that automates both our payments out and credits in and serves to streamline our personal monthly reconciliations of cash flows. With the advent of online shopping, a shift has occurred in how we shop. Instead of visiting a mall, we take time out of our work week to shop online, making more efficient use of our time and removing the hassle of lugging our purchases around with us, with free or low-cost home delivery services. Another example: in most cities these days we rarely hail a taxi; instead, we "call" an Uber or Lyft car to pick us up at a determined spot and time that we electronically order through our mobile phones. Some of these new practices take time to learn and get used to, but often, with some practice, we find they serve us better, saving us time, money, and effort. (I offer a few caveats to these new "processes" we so quickly adopt, including our love of Uber/Lyft. Flip to Chapter 14 to read more.)

Financial Investments

When it comes to pursuing deep sustainability, it's necessary to make financial investments in technologies that support better efficiency and optimize resource use. We also need to consider investments to help us transition away from fossil fuel use toward renewables, so that our use of electricity to light, heat, and cool our homes and power our electronics and vehicles is emission-less, as much as humanly possible.

Efficiency means improving the mechanisms we use so that we need less of something to achieve the same outcome. An example we know well is high-efficiency (HE) clothing washers. Front-loading washing machines are an upgrade to traditional washing machines. The technology—the internal mechanism used to wash our clothes—allows us to use energy and water more efficiently. HE washers use eighty percent less water than traditional washing machines.

To optimize is to automate or systematize a process so that peak efficiency, productivity, and use can be realized. Financial investments in technologies that optimize the way we use resources are hugely impactful. Think about a lawn irrigation system for new trees and bushes just planted. Here's an example that may be familiar to you.

You just spent good money landscaping your home. You'd like to ensure your plants don't wither and die in the heat of summer. So, you decide to invest in an irrigation system. You reckon, rightly, that the upfront cost of the lawn irrigation pays for itself in just a year's time because it's a good insurance policy against dead plants and it takes the burden off you remembering when you should water the plants, how often, and by what means.

Now, that irrigation system can be enhanced with additional technology by attaching it to a GPS that monitors weather fluctuations in the area where you live. The GPS is a "smart" application that dynamically determines when the irrigation system should operate; in this case, when to flow water to the plants. On rainy days, the irrigation system remains dormant. On hot, sunny days, the GPS will "tell" the system to flow water to your plants for a period of time that appropriately hydrates your plants given the temperature and humidity calculated by the system. Your irrigation system just got optimized.

Now, think about the case for replacing your incandescent light bulbs with LED ones. Transitioning to LED bulbs in your home solves for both efficiency and optimization goals. LED is a technology that uses energy more efficiently, requiring just ten percent of what incandescents need, and optimizes the life of bulbs, which typically have lifespans between three and five years, versus months with the old Edison invention.

Lastly, we must consider investments that support ours and the rest of humanity's transition to emissions-free energy, otherwise known as renewables. Think electric vehicles, rooftop solar panels, solar stoves, and geothermal loop systems that harness Earth's core heat to warm our homes (read more about this in Chapter 8). These are technologies we need to consider investing in to support deep reductions in our personal contributions to climate change.

New technologies originate to replace or substitute products or processes that are less efficient or more harmful to the environment. All require some upfront investment. Many are affordable, especially if federal and state subsidies are considered.

These three change considerations will determine the size of sustainability measures you will want to pursue: small, medium, or large. Size refers to both the size of the impact the action will have on reducing our carbon contributions to climate change, as well as the amount of effort and resources that implementing a sustainability measure will require from you.

Let's rename these changes and refer to them as levers we can "pull." When it comes to determining which sustainability measures to pursue, you will need to evaluate the following:

Lever #1: Level of behavior change acceptable to you

Lever #2: Level of process change you are willing to adopt to cement new behaviors into habits

Lever #3: Level of financial investment needed to successfully implement a sustainability measure

Let's delve into each in turn.

The Behavior Lever

Behavior changes are not easy to implement. We all have made sweeping statements in our lives about how we are going to stop doing something and, instead, pursue a new, healthier habit. Here are a few behavior change statements that may be familiar to you:

- I'm going to go to bed earlier during the weekdays so I can get a better night's sleep.

- I'm going to drink wine only on the weekends.

- I'm going to work out five days a week.

- I'm going to keep my grocery spending to $300 every week.

- I'm going to stop smoking.

Now, the first step to making any change is to recognize what you want to change or what you want to do differently. This is where we all start. The problem is, just saying something does not make it reality. Changing ingrained, repetitive, even subconscious behaviors is difficult. Behaviors take time to change. We have to be consciously aware of how we move ourselves from the old to the new. Behaviors have to be performed repeatedly. We need to retrain our mind, our body, our psyche. And we need to meet with some form of success to cement the behavior into habit.

The Process Lever

This is where you develop new processes that you'll rely on to ensure your behavior change declaration will be followed and enacted. That doesn't mean there won't be hiccups along the way to cementing a new behavior, but a process for getting you there has to be in place for you to meet with success. Behavior changes and processes to support those changes go hand in hand. Their importance cannot be overstated when it comes to pursuing sustainable action.

In my work performing carbon inventories for companies, I help businesses set carbon reduction targets by using the SMART goal framework. SMART stands for

S: Specific—Set specific goals that lead to action.

M: Measurable—Progress toward the goal is quantifiable.

A: Achievable—Ensure that goals set are met and/or can be completed.

R: Relevant—Make sure you know what you are trying to accomplish.

T: Time-bound—The goal is implemented in the time desired.

Below is a process example for one of the previously stated desired behavior changes. I will use the SMART goal framework to develop a process roadmap to meet with the behavioral goal.

Example: I'm going to go to bed earlier during the weekdays so I can get a better night's sleep.

S: I will go to bed, lights out, by 10 pm Monday to Thursday.

M: The kids' routine is starting to shift to an earlier and more reliable bedtime and lights-out program. Reading for twenty minutes before my goal bedtime relaxes me and sets me up to sleep soundly.

A: I can achieve my goal if I follow this schedule:

1 The family eats by 6:30 pm.
2 Dinner clean-up is completed by 7 pm.
3 Kids get one hour of screen time before bedtime routines.
4 Kids finish baths/showers and teeth-brushing by 8:30 pm.
5 Bedtime reading and goodnight rituals are complete by 9 pm.
6 I have forty minutes to watch news, read, and prepare myself for bed.
7 Lights out by 10 pm.

R: I know I need a solid eight hours to feel good and have productive workdays.

T: I will give myself two weeks to achieve my goal of a 10 pm bedtime.

The Financial Investment Lever

Not all but many sustainability measures will require some upfront financial investment. Some will be of minimal cost; others will demand a more significant commitment of financial resources.

Purchasing a compost bin for your kitchen is arguably a minimal financial cost. Installing a geothermal system to heat your home and water is a larger financial investment that requires planning and hiring of experts to complete the installation work. Here, you need to assess for yourself what sustainability measures you are willing to invest in because they are important to you and they fall within your financial capabilities.

There is no shame in admitting that you are not pursuing or prioritizing a sustainable action because it's not in your budget or the payoff is not sufficiently quick or large enough. We all have to make choices that fit our values and our financial situations. The good news about sustainability is that some of the most impactful measures do not cost a significant amount of money.

Below is a mapping of behavior and process changes, as well as the likely financial investment required, to pursue several sustainability measures. Note that I've designated how big each of the example measures will be, considering the level of effort and personal cost needed to implement them.

Sustainability Measure	Behavior Changes	Process Changes	Financial Investment	Size of Sustainability Impact
Use cold-water setting on dishwasher	Yes— one time	No	No	Small

Sustainability Measure	Behavior Changes	Process Changes	Financial Investment	Size of Sustainability Impact
Flush home toilets every other trip to bathroom	Yes— every time	Yes Actively not flush every time Close seat cover Enlist family participation	No	Medium
Purchase LED bulbs	Yes— ongoing	Yes Research LED bulbs desired for each room/activity application Purchase bulbs Replace all incandescents	Yes New bulb purchases	Large

From the change mapping above, you can develop a decision framework to determine how much personal change and investment is comfortable for you. This would be customized to your personal preferences, your tolerance for change, and the level of sustainability impact you want to pursue. Here's an example:

Sustainability Measure	Behavior Changes	Process Changes	Amount of Financial Investment
Reduce plastic wrap use	Will not stop using Try to adopt alternatives to plastic wrap	Rely on existing Tupperware with lids Try waxed cotton wraps as a substitute	No more than $20

Sustainability Measure	Behavior Changes	Process Changes	Amount of Financial Investment
Upgrade clothing washer and dryer to HE appliances	Wash clothes only with full loads Wash loads on tap water setting	Commit to reducing clothing washes to three times per week	No more than $1,200
Reduce animal meat consumption	Eat no animal meat for lunches	Purchase no lunch meats. Make or buy plant-based protein soups Adopt hearty green, grain, and vegetable-based salads.	None

"Just Right" Sustainability Measures

Remember the story of Goldilocks and the three bears? A little girl wanders into the house of a family of three bears: a mama, daddy, and baby bear. She ventures into the kitchen and tries a taste of each of three bowls of porridge. One's too hot and one's too cold, but one is "just right," and she eats it all up.

What does Goldilocks have to do with you and sustainability? It's a metaphor for trying on for size, so to speak, sustainability measures to see if they work for you. You might think you're really going to dig not using plastic sandwich bags or committing to becoming a vegan. Once you've made the commitment, you find out that for some things, like storing pastry dough in the freezer, for example, a plastic Ziploc bag is best. Or, eating vegan may be making you anemic and feeling lethargic. You have to reassess and adjust the sustainability measures you've put in place to fit your values and your lifestyle.

The story of the three bears could play out somewhat differently. You could decide that you are going to first commit to eating less meat. In actuality, that may mean that you have made a conscious choice to not eat meat during breakfast and lunch meals. You find after a couple of months that not eating meat feels really good to your body and the effort has been easy for you. You decide to rev up your "no eating meat" commitment and transition to being a pescatarian or a vegetarian.

Another example could be that you want to see if you can use your car less each week. You first decide to commute once a week to work. That commitment transitions to commuting two to three times per week. After a period of time, you decide that because your round trip to work is less than ten miles, you are going to purchase an electric bike to commute to work. Your first set of commitments ramped up after a period of trial and adjustment. They worked, and you got to a point where escalating—deepening—your sustainability commitments felt right and was in line with and reinforced your well-being, livelihood, and sense of purpose.

Deciding on Your Commitment Level

We all need to decide what level of commitment to sustainability feels right to us and is doable right now. As you've seen, commitments can be small, medium, or large in size.

Small measures have less of an impact on reducing carbon emissions than large ones, but both have beneficial effects. Driving a hybrid versus an EV has less of an impact on carbon emission reductions, but both are more beneficial than blind loyalty to a combustion-engine vehicle. The same goes for skipping meat in a meal once a week versus eating no meat; both are beneficial, but the latter has a greater impact on reducing carbon emissions throughout the entire food chain.

Each scale of action requires a change in your approach to daily activities and, in some cases, a financial investment to implement sustainable measures that are lasting.

In the next chapter, I will introduce you to impact categories, which chunk and parcel sustainability measures into specific areas of your life. If you don't own a house, home sustainability measures may not be where you focus your efforts. Don't own a car? Then you can skip that impact category and focus on more relevant categories, like food and trash.

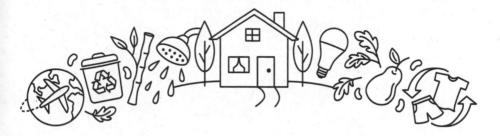

4

....

Getting Curious about Carbon

One of the biggest
obstacles to making a
start on climate change
is that it has become
a cliché before it has
even been understood.

TIM FLANNERY, *The Weather Makers*

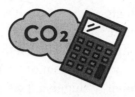

I F YOU remember your chemistry class in high school or college, carbon (C) was just one of the 118 elements on the periodic table you likely memorized and then promptly forgot. Carbon is naturally occurring in nature. If you received an engagement ring from or purchased one for your beloved and the stone is of the crystal-clear variety—a diamond—you own carbon. If you like to swat yellow balls over a low green fence with a partner using a graphite racket, you know carbon.

Carbon combines with oxygen to form carbon dioxide (CO_2), a molecule that we expel when we breathe, and that trees and plants absorb to grow. This process of expelling and absorbing is a beautiful system that supports human and non-human life on Earth.

Fossil fuels are made up of carbon. Oil, gas, and coal are hydrocarbons, a combination of hydrogen and carbon. Burning these fuels, as we do, for energy, electricity, and making products sends a whole heck of a lot of CO_2 into the air, along with many other noxious, not-so-good-for-you, invisible chemicals like carbon monoxide (CO), sulfur dioxide (SO_2), nitrogen dioxide (NO_2), methane (CH_4), and substances grouped into a category known as volatile organic compounds (VOCs). Most of these chemicals pollute the air we breathe. They also happen to heat up the air and, thus, the planet. Because we burn so much fossil fuel all the time across the globe, we've created climate change.

We know better, but energy from burning fossil fuels is so powerful, we have a hard time weaning ourselves. All of our systems for the last two hundred years have been built to dig up, refine, ship, and burn fossil fuels efficiently and relatively cheaply. Our entrenched infrastructure—underground pipelines, national railroad systems, central utility grids—and continued federal subsidies to the coal, oil, and gas industries make our transition to better-for-the-world renewable energy sluggish. Unfortunately, fossil fuels are great until they're not.

The burning of fossil fuels by humans has created climate change. These energy sources continue to increase global warming. They are exacerbating the impacts we are experiencing in the form of extreme weather events. Fossil fuels have got to go bye-bye.

Our Carbon Contributions

As individuals, we can't directly change whether our federal government, our state, or our city stops using fossil fuels. But we can influence them for sure. The same goes for companies that manufacture products for individual consumption. You can't prevent any one company from not using natural gas to heat their corporate offices, but you can influence them to move away from fossil fuels toward a renewable source of energy. You persuade by how and what you buy. You persuade by being vocal and asking entities you need and rely on to adopt a better way. You start by understanding what you control and where your efforts have the biggest impact on your life.

Let me give you a quick primer on personal carbon footprints. A carbon footprint is a summary of all the greenhouse gas (GHG) emissions, generically referred to as "carbon," that one person or a group of people, say a family, emits into the atmosphere. We live, so we do. If activities that we perform or purchases that we make use fossil fuels either indirectly or directly, those activities and purchases can be thrown into the "negative impact" bin.

So what is direct and indirect?

Direct carbon emissions are simple: direct activity is what you physically do, directly, that contributes to your personal carbon contributions. You purchase gas to run your car. When you turn your car on or "ignite" the engine that runs on gas, that is direct activity. Another example is the energy source we use to turn on the lights in our home. If that source is some non-zero percentage from fossil fuel, that's a direct link.

Indirect carbon emissions are harder to determine sometimes, but they are everywhere in your life. If you use plastic bags or plastic containers, that is an indirect consumption of fossil fuel. If you buy a pair of Supplex yoga pants, that's an indirect consumption of fossil fuel. If you buy a LEGO *Star Wars: The Mandalorian* set for your son, that is an indirect consumption of fossil fuel.

Other than your utility bill and the gas you buy for your automobile, most of your carbon footprint is made up of indirect sources. That can get tricky, but I'm here to help give you a framework for thinking about how to categorize activities that indirectly contribute to your carbon footprint so that you can start influencing and controlling reductions in both those indirect contributions and your direct ones as well.

Personal Carbon Footprints: What Are They?

We've gotta understand that we need to reduce our individual carbon footprints. They are too high. It's because we buy so many things made from fossil fuels.

Economists tend to refer to each individual in per capita terms. Per capita just means "for each person."

An average American emits 15.56 metric tons of CO_2 annually.[1] Nearly thirty percent (4.7 metric tons) of that comes from using combustion-engine cars.[2]

OK, but how can you make sense of that 15.56 metric tons of "carbon"? What does it mean to you? Probably not much right now. How big or small is that number? How do Americans compare to other "average" individuals who live in Europe, Asia, Africa, and Latin America?

Comparisons are useful when we're trying to wrap our head around a number and a metric we don't use anywhere in our daily life. We don't set our water usage to metric tons. We don't measure our flour and sugar in metric tons when we're cooking. Metric tons is an abstract measurement that we cannot visualize. But let's compare amounts with other average individuals across the globe.

Here is a hand-selected list of countries that are highly developed or considered fast-developing countries, and their average per capita metric ton (MT) of carbon, ranked from lowest to highest:[3]

Kenya: 0.34 MT
India: 1.92 MT
Brazil: 2.23 MT
Thailand: 3.93 MT
Sweden: 4.54 MT
France: 4.6 MT
Turkey: 4.63 MT
United Kingdom: 5.59 MT
Denmark: 6.66 MT
China: 8.12 MT
Germany: 9.47 MT
Netherlands: 9.61 MT
United States: 15.56 MT
Saudi Arabia: 16.01 MT
Australia: 17.22 MT
Canada: 18.62 MT
United Arab Emirates: 23.60 MT

You might be thinking after scanning the list, *Phew, the average American is not the* most *(negatively) impactful to the planet*. And you'd be right. Per capita—each person on average—in Canada and Australia contributes more than any one American does. Take a look at the United Arab Emirates. Its average citizen contributes to climate change just over fifty percent more than an average American does.

The comparisons are helpful, but they don't give us the complete picture. America is home to more than 331 million people. The populations of Canada (38 million), Australia (25 million), and the UAE (around 10 million) combined total 73 million people, just twenty-two percent of all the people in the US. Said another way, because of how many of us there are, Americans contribute 4.5 times more to climate change than the top three countries together.

Clearly, the US has near-equivalent industries and economies to that of the European Union members, and most of the EU has dramatically lower CO_2 emission rates than the US. It should be noted that less developed countries, such as those in Southeast Asia and Africa, have extremely low per capita emission rates, with Australia (and New Zealand) and the more developed Middle East nations out-emitting the US by a significant margin. The takeaway? The US is not the worst-emitting nation on a per person basis, but we are a force to be reckoned with, since our population is large and growing and we have the means in our grasp to dramatically lower our per capita CO_2 annual emissions levels.

There is another story to be told here. Go back and scan the list once more. Make a mental note of the total metric tons per capita for Denmark, the Netherlands, and Germany: 6.66, 9.61, and 9.47 metric tons per capita. The Denmark number is close to one-third of the US total.

No one can argue that life in Denmark, the Netherlands, or Germany is not comfortable and good. Denmark is often rated the world's happiest country. The Netherlands consistently rates its citizens as highly satisfied with work and life, and Dutch kids are rated the happiest in Europe.[4] Germany by all measures has a strong, thriving economy that provides opportunity and financial security to its citizens. These countries and their people are flourishing. There's that word again: flourishing.

Let's look at the UK for a minute. On average, individuals in the UK reduced their annual CO_2 emission rates by more than thirty-eight percent over a ten-year span (2006 to 2016), close to a four percent carbon reduction annually.[5] If we did something similar to what we see in the UK, here's what our individual carbon footprints could look like:

A thirty percent carbon reduction: 10.89 metric tons emitted
A fifty percent carbon reduction: 7.78 metric tons emitted

And because you always need a moon-shot goal in your life:

An eighty percent carbon reduction: 3.11 metric tons of CO_2 emitted

Americans could get themselves—each of us—down to below Thailand levels over the course of ten years by making incremental tweaks to our activities and by being mindful of how and what we buy. C'mon! That's cool. And totally doable.

Do you want to know how? Start pursuing sustainability in your own life.

Last Thoughts on Carbon

I don't want you to think about your carbon footprint. I want you to think about sustainability measures you can take that align with your personal values and that fit into your life in such a way that they become natural, everyday habits. I want you to equate sustainable actions with fun, freedom, choice, and innovation. Because when you get right down to it, choosing sustainable behaviors, making sustainable choices, and pursuing sustainable options involves creativity, new technical solutions, and authenticity. There is no one right way to be sustainable. We all have personal agency. I want you to feel empowered to make a plan that works for you and serves you.

Remember, sustainability is not a sacrifice. It's a change in lifestyle that allows you to flourish.

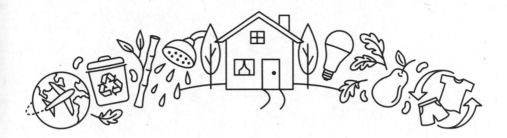

5
....

Bias to
Action

The first step binds one to the second.

FRENCH PROVERB

ALTHOUGH HUMANS consider themselves the "big kahunas" among the species that inhabit Earth, our fates are intimately tied to the productivity, diversity, and health of all the other non-human life that makes up this world. Our health is supported by an abundance of diversity. One good example of this truth is what happens when gene pools become too homogenous or similar. The known risk of inbreeding is an increased propensity for rare diseases and deformity in offspring. DNA and organisms thrive in highly diverse ecosystems. Greater diversity breeds healthfulness. By planting a rich, diverse diet of grains, fruits, and vegetables—from seeds that are native to local regions—biodiverse farming supports the health and vitality of whole communities in meaningful, dynamic ways. Good health increases our happiness and supports our productivity. Our livelihoods and economies are dependent on human productivity. This virtuous cycle of diversity breeding health that supports productivity is the unseen DNA of our ecosystem. Humans are dependent upon these interconnected systems.

When it comes to climate change, we are all affected. I call it an equal opportunity impactor. Texans near the shores of the Gulf of Mexico have been brutalized by hurricanes and flooding. Florida's Key West is literally sinking along with its historic houses. Nearly the whole of California is on fire ... all year long.

Personal sustainability is about realizing that although these things—extreme weather impacts—are happening across the US and to other people and communities, they may soon enough come to your city or town and directly affect your life and that of your family. Taking sustainable action is about pitching in to support the human system of living, where and how you can. It's about raising your hand and declaring, "I care."

Sustainability measures, whether you can see their effects or not, help support biodiversity in your local community, build productivity into your water systems and soils, and maintain and grow the health of your land, water, and air for the benefit of individuals like you, as well as our non-human "friends." Your sustainability actions are not isolated. They, together with others' actions, form a potent brew in supporting our planet's "operating" system. Consider the butterfly effect, a principle from chaos theory: small things (such as actions, behaviors, and decisions) occurring somewhere in a complex system (such as planet Earth) are capable of having dramatic impacts on or within the system. Of course, you are aiming for positive impacts, not detrimental ones. Sustainability measures are your ticket to affecting the climate system in beneficial ways.

A story that aired on *60 Minutes*, the CBS Sunday evening news show, is an effective thought piece on the value of personal sustainability. Steve Kroft opened his segment by introducing the Isle of Eigg, a small island off the coast of Scotland, to viewers. The island is home to just one hundred residents, not all of whom are of Scottish descent. It is a small chunk of land, just three miles wide by six miles long. The Isle of Eigg is essentially an egalitarian society: owned and run by its inhabitants. There is no formal local government to name.

Although the island is incredibly beautiful, it lacks most natural resources. Most of the island's fuel for vehicles and basic food supplies have to be shipped in by boat, and those boats don't come frequently. Perhaps because of the nature of its dependencies and its lack of resource options, the residents of Eigg implemented a progressive idea: powering nearly one hundred percent of the island with renewable energy using a mix of wind, solar, and hydroelectric power. Eigg has become a global model for how to implement a highly workable distributed energy system that doesn't contribute to climate change. Hence how it found itself showcased on *60 Minutes*.

The Eigg segment, though, is about much more than an economy and a way of life run on renewable energy. It's a microcosm of how to think about self, community, and surviving in order to thrive in an environment that is incredibly beautiful and valued by individuals but has limited resources. Kroft mused that "to survive, they have to *rely on* each other, *look after* each other, and *put up with* each other. The island is too small for feuds or lingering resentments."[1] Near the end of the piece, one of the saltier characters who doubles as a cab driver on the island stated his belief that Eigg residents are "more evolved." Kroft summed up his observations about the island and its people: "To live here you have to be resilient, self-sufficient, and patient."

We are all living on an island. It's called Earth. It is the only planet in the Milky Way that supports human life and the fecundity of other life as we know it. Earth is our Isle of Eigg. It is beautiful. We cherish it. The planet is fertile, yes, but finite in its resources.

Think big. Bigger than yourself, your family, your neighborhood, and your state. Think of yourself in a broader context: one species among millions seeking to thrive on another living organism—Earth. If you can support the planet to function better in the ways you are able, every species inherently benefits from your actions.

You should also think of yourself as being in a process of evolving your thinking about what is sustainable, why it is important, and how to incorporate sustainability into your life. So too, you should view your realm of influence to include your broader community: seek to build yours and others' capacities while bearing with others as they try, tinker, and refine their sustainable actions.

The goal of personal sustainability is to be resilient—to bend but not break—in the face of climate change's extreme weather impacts. Personal sustainability is about empowering yourself to be an agent of change; to be self-sufficient in taking action. And critically, capacity building of sustainability measures takes time, just like stopping and reversing climate change will take time. We are learning a new way of living, and embracing a lifestyle that is joyful, light, vibrant, and healthy. Be patient with yourself.

You could amend Kroft's ending thought about the Isle of Eigg by making an affirmative statement for yourself: To live sustainably on Earth, I have to be resilient, self-sufficient, and patient.

part two

NOURISHING SEEDS

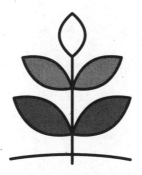

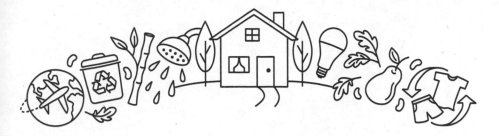

6
....

Living Lightly, Living Well

It's because of the people who
are working toward sustainability...
that I know how quickly the decision
to go that direction, though it may
start out with a feeling of sacrifice,
turns into a lifetime of rejoicing.

DONELLA H. MEADOWS

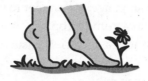

HAVE YOU watched *Bee Movie*? It's a 2007 film that stars Jerry Seinfeld, Matthew Broderick, Renée Zellweger, and my always-favorite, John Goodman. It's a charming piece of animation. It's about bees, a florist, and the human race. The plot line involves one college-educated worker bee, played by Seinfeld, who is fed up with the prospect of a life of work making honey, suing humans, successfully, so they will stop eating and profiting from the sale of bees' honey. With that bit of species win, bees take a holiday and stop pollinating the world and, of course, making honey for humans. The downside? The world begins to die.

The great, mostly small pollinators of the world—ants, bats, bees, beetles, birds, butterflies, flies, moths, and wasps—are responsible for ensuring that more than eighty percent of the world's flowering plants reproduce.[1] Our health and nutrition depend on an ecosystem we mostly take for granted. Without bees, butterflies, and birds, we'd see our gorgeous green and blue planet turn brown. No more apples, pears, berries, nuts, squashes, pumpkins, watermelons, cucumbers, and more. Most fruits or vegetables with a nut or seed require some kind of pollinator to help the plants bear fruit.

When we hear about planting native trees and plants and conversations about eradicating "invasives," the point is a sharp one. Native plants support local pollinators to sustain themselves and thrive. Invasives are a little like a foreign language: they are hard for species to understand. They don't know what they are and what to do with them because they are foreign and, thus, different. The pollinators of the world aren't attracted to them; plants and pollinators don't speak the same language. It's similar to when the first settlers arrived in New England from Europe in 1620. They didn't know what was native to America and tried unsuccessfully to plant and grow staples from the Old World: rye, barley, and wheat and a variety of English garden vegetables.

The first settlers learned which plants would survive and bear fruit from the local Native Americans, the Wampanoag. The settlers were taught how to grow the "Three Sisters" crops: corn, squash, and beans. These plants, native to America, grew well as a team in poor, sandy soils that didn't retain nutrients or water well. Without the benefit of the Native Americans who shared their knowledge of plants in America, the pilgrims would have perished.

Knowledge is a powerful tool for change. For the American pilgrims, it was literally life-giving. Without the sharing of knowledge on the importance of sustainability, many of us wouldn't know what is possible, probable, and doable.

I'm taking a tiny leap here to state, unequivocally, that all of us want to live in a world that supports us and is supported in return. We want to do the right thing, the best thing, the sustainable thing that will allow us to live well on this earth and shepherd its natural resources along safely and abundantly to our kids and, again, to their kids. That means we fundamentally care about taking care of the planet. Sharing sustainability knowledge within and among our communities is the key ingredient for making these ideas living and breathing priorities.

Managing Our Impact

Everything we do has an impact on the world. That impact can be positive, like when we coach our kid's soccer team. We are teaching new skills and universal life lessons. We are promoting teamwork—and how it feels to work, win, and lose together. We are keeping kids active, enjoying physical activity in the natural environment. From one act, many positive impacts and ripple effects are produced.

Impacts can also be negative. It could be as simple as walking past a piece of litter, say an empty Doritos bag. You register it but don't pick it up. It's not yours or your concern, you say to yourself. That plastic bag is not biodegradable. It will float and glide until it stops somewhere in a bush or stand of trees if not picked up. Over time, it may get buried under dirt or ingested by a bird or other wild animal. Because plastic is made from petroleum and natural gas, it's toxic to soils and to animals. It pollutes.

One of my favorite Jivamukti yoga teachers in NYC, Matt, used to ask us to be conscious about doing at least one positive thing a day. He'd tell us what he did, which usually involved trash. He'd say, "If you're walking down the street and see a piece of trash, pick it up and put it in a waste bin. Every time you see a piece of trash, repeat the process. It doesn't take too much effort. The very act cleans up the street, and you can lay claim to performing a positive act."

Some impacts are neutral on the environment. It feels weird saying that, but it's true. Walking and biking are perfect examples. They are great for us both mentally and physically. For the earth, it's a shrug. And that's saying something!

Here's the thing. We have to eat, sleep, move, and work. We have to perform all the activities required in order for us to keep on living, working, and progressing. To live sustainably doesn't mean to stop living or to limit how we live. We're setting our goal on flourishing, right? Living sustainably requires us to decipher what impacts our living and all the activities that are rolled into that endeavor have on the broader world around us.

Are you able to assess what activities, decisions, and purchases have a negative, positive, or neutral impact on the planet? We need to group our personal activities into categories that make sense and are easy to remember. I call them impact categories. By categorizing your activities, you will be able to mine jewels of sustainability that are valuable and meaningful to you, and thus can be maintained.

Impact Category #1: Transportation

One of the largest areas under our direct control is how we get from our house to where we need to be and back, whether that be work, the kids' schools, the gym, or the grocery store. All of the choices you make on how you travel and by what mode fall into this category, including

- what type of automobile you drive;
- how often it is used;
- what distance needs to be completed;
- what fuel or energy that vehicle requires; and
- whether you use other forms of transportation for your everyday activities.

The transportation category makes up one-third of all our personal emissions that contribute to climate change. Whatever decisions we make here have an outsized influence on our personal sustainability.

Impact Category #2: Energy

This category includes choices such as what energy type you use to heat and cool your home and water, how you light your home, what energy source you use to cook, and how you power your personal electronic devices.

Impact Category #3: Home and Property

This category involves the building where you live, whether owned or rented, and how it is constructed, including roof and insulation choices. It also includes any land or property on which your home sits or abuts. In this category, I will ask you to consider the size of your home, its heating and cooling systems, and where it is located, as well as renovation considerations, especially if you are the owner or potential buyer of an existing home.

Impact Category #4: Food

This category is a big one, up there with transportation. Our industrial agriculture system for growing food makes up more than thirty percent of global carbon emissions. In America, that carbon contribution notches down to twenty percent of the country's total. What you decide to eat and how much can have a big impact—positive or negative—on global sustainability. There are some juicy nuggets of opportunity in this category: small changes that make a big carbon impact. We are going to discuss local versus industrial, GMOs, antibiotics and steroids, and alternatives to animal and fish protein.

Impact Category #5: Material Goods

This is another category where huge sustainability strides can be made. Why, you may ask? Because everything we buy has a story to be told. And like most post–Industrial Revolution stories, they are filled, baked, and then glazed with fossil fuels. We are going to talk about natural and recycled materials in clothing, footwear, furniture, and homewares.

Impact Category #6: Water

Water is a precious, vulnerable resource, and scarcity is a real concern here in the US, where we turn on the taps without worry and it flows freely. Thinking about the different "types" of water—blue, gray, green, and black—can reveal opportunities for conservation. This category includes how we use water, how it is delivered to us, what conservation measures we can put in place, and how we can capture water that falls from the sky and use or divert it well.

Impact Category #7: Trash

Here's the short take on this category: trash isn't waste if we can look at it just a little bit differently. I'm going to seek to apply Otto Scharmer's Theory U framework to this category and ask you to shift how you view trash, not as waste but as valuable material. Scharmer's Theory U asks individuals to build their capacity for solving human problems by harnessing an ecosystem (versus egocentric) perspective. By understanding the lifespan of materials and allocating them in appropriate ways, we can work toward eliminating waste from the planet.

IN THE previous pages I've listed seven impact categories. These are all areas under your control in some way, shape, or form. You have the ability to make changes—small, medium, and large—in how you buy and the activities you pursue that involve these categories. By pursuing sustainability measures within each, you grow your positive and neutralize your negative impacts on the earth.

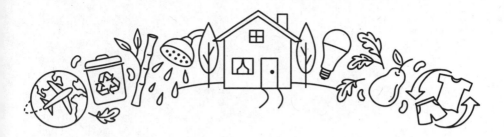

7
....

Transportation

In order to have
clean air in cities, you
have to go electric.

ELON MUSK

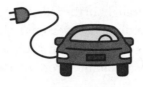

THE TRANSPORTATION impact category kicks off first before all others because it has the potential to decrease your personal contributions to climate change by thirty percent. Especially if you currently drive a combustion-engine vehicle to commute to work or zip around town to complete your household errands. This category is an area rife with opportunity to rethink how we go about getting life done.

My Superiority Complex

Hey, I'm not ashamed to admit it. It's a delight to drive an electric vehicle (EV). I became an owner of a leased BMW i3 in the spring of 2019. I had spent the previous three years persuading my husband that we should purchase an EV. I needed one, desperately. I felt it to be the most responsible thing I could do as an individual and one well within my grasp to accomplish.

A half year earlier, in October 2018, the United Nations Intergovernmental Panel on Climate Change (IPCC) published a special report on global warming.[1] Among the many revelatory predictions from its climate scenarios, one stuck out: our carbon emissions budgets need radical alteration. One of the biggest and easiest levers for reducing mine (and others') is rethinking by what mechanism I move myself around. And when I say mechanism, I mean what mode of transport to use in my daily commuting life.

I found myself distraught in the fall of 2018. I knew the statistic: almost a third of an individual's personal carbon footprint comes from GHG emissions combusted by their automobile. Why was I, of all people—a sustainability professional—still driving a gas-combusting vehicle?

Primacy here in the US is placed on driving. Particularly, driving alone and autonomously, embodying the idea of being masters of our domain. But, at what cost? Driving combustion-engine automobiles pollutes our air and makes people sick. Anyone who holds a job in a decently sized city knows the particular hell of commuting traffic. We inch along, hurrying up to keep at a crawl, to inevitably arrive at work stressed and frustrated by how long our commute took.

At one point in my tenure at XM Satellite Radio, I was waking up at four in the morning to jump in my car thirty minutes later in an effort to reduce the congested commute that awaited me on Route 66 and Interstate 495 (the Capital Beltway)—a distance of thirty-four miles—from two and a half hours to one and a half hours. I was a basket case when I arrived at work, often needing to sneak a quick nap in around 6:30 am before the workday began.

Today, I don't find myself driving very much. For the last four years, I've averaged about three miles of driving a day; 1,100 a year. My auto insurance provider loves me (and rewards me) for that low level of driving. I reside in the northwest hills of downtown Portland. My kids' elementary school is less than a mile from my home. Most everything I need to do on a daily basis—grocery shop, pick up supplies at the pharmacy, grab an afternoon coffee, and withdraw money from my bank—is accessible within a two-mile radius of my house. I do need a car for some key activities with my kids, but I don't need to drive most days.

And so, I became one of those people: an EV owner and driver.

It's a joy to drive. It's so zippy. You can gun the accelerator and there's no lag to pick up speed. It's super stealthy. I often feel like a creeper to pedestrians. Because no sound comes from the engine of the i3—more like a low, soft hum—people often don't perceive I'm there, on the road.

I just dig my EV's regenerative brakes. It's become a game I play with myself: how soon before I make a turn do I release my foot from the accelerator to slow down to the right speed to avoid a brake tap in order to execute a smooth turn. Regenerative brakes automatically slow a car down once the accelerator is released. Cooler still, the EV braking system captures "otherwise-wasted kinetic energy" and converts it to electricity by recharging the car's battery.[2] The driver dashboard panel displays by how much the battery is getting recharged. A favorite game I have is to clock how much charge my EV has at the start of any vehicle trip, then see whether I can maintain the same charge—or better, increase it (without plugging into a charging station)—by the time I get home, just by gaming the use of my regenerative brakes.

Yes, I'm going to admit it. In the first couple of months driving my EV around town and on longer routes involving multi-lane highways, I'd look out across the sea of combustion-engine vehicles and wonder, with not a small amount of dismay, why in the world more people haven't gotten on the EV bandwagon. Why were so many people still driving their fossil-fuel-combusting, greenhouse-gas-emitting, smog-producing automobiles?

I felt this swelling sense of righteousness that I had forced my own hand and done the right thing. I knew that the very act of my driving was doing nothing detrimental to the environment. It was a personal exhale. OK, I kept thinking, *This is what it feels like to act responsibly and do right by the planet!* I felt good about myself. And yes, somewhat abashedly now, I felt an early sense of superiority to the combustion-engine automobile drivers sharing the roads with me.

My righteousness and sense of superiority have waned. Now, I just feel deep relief that I'm not contributing to climate change while driving. Today, I am adamant about catalyzing and progressing a societal transition to zero-carbon transporting. With eyes wide open, I view myself as an example-setter, one among many growing hundreds of thousands of individuals here in the US who show their commitment to climate change mitigation by the very act of driving an EV. It's a singular commitment that turns into a personal ethos that permeates a community to live sustainably. As the old saying goes, "Actions speak louder than words."

Walking and Biking Are Cool

Why must we persist in our lowly view of bipedal and two-wheeled modes of transportation?

Walking

Commuting by walking is a New York state of mind in Manhattan. I calculated my commute from my apartment to my work building according to how long it took me to stride across five and a half avenues and up six blocks on foot. It took me twenty-one minutes to walk a mile across to the east side of the island and uptown to the Flatiron District from the neighborhood of Chelsea. In heels. If I quickened my pace, I could arrive in eighteen minutes, especially if I crossed through Madison Square Park, which was under construction at the time and empty of lingering pedestrians.

I remember meeting my first boss, Ann Duffy, when I took a job at Time Inc. She and I would grab lunch those first few months together, and she never stopped for a streetlight. She timed her steps so that if crossing a street was unavailable in one direction, she'd transfer by foot to the opposite side of the block so she could catch the "Pedestrian Walking" sign allowing individuals the right of way in front of cars. Ann would bolt left and forward, right and forward, navigating the avenues and streets until she met with her destination in the most efficient bipedal means I had experienced to date.

New Yorkers know how to buy shoes for walking. I quickly learned to always pack my "destination" shoes in my big purse duffel. Your feet are for walking. I, like most of my fellow Gotham dwellers, typically averaged three to five miles of walking daily on weekdays and eight to ten miles on the weekends, when it was necessary to perform errands, meet friends, exercise, and fit in some fun during off-work hours, all on foot.

Walking is a built-in exercise routine. The health guidelines set by the US Department of Health and Human Services recommend thirty minutes of walking five times a week.[3] One walk to your local grocery store will check that requirement off your weekly exercise checklist.

Have you ever noticed that getting to take a walk allows your mind to think creatively, but also your shoulders to relax and your breath to deepen? It does for me. It takes about twenty minutes before I start feeling mentally lighter, which translates into a happier and psychologically healthier me. Daily walks these days, as a professional working woman and a mother of two kids, give me the ability to successfully transition out of the stresses of the workday into family time, fully present and calm.

Did I tire of walking in New York sometimes? Yes, I did. That's when I'd hop on the buses that traverse the city north and south, east and west. But generally, I enjoyed walking. It kept me fit and active, breathing in fresh air, communing physically with the world. So, yes, in NYC, walking was a state of mind. In other parts of the country, walking can be a way of life. Walking is a clean and healthy mode of transportation, with the added benefit of recalibrating your zinging brain back to a place where being fully present is objectively doable again.

Biking

For most of the last century, bikes were relegated for use either recreationally or competitively. There wasn't much in between. Biking as a mode of common transport is going through a radical transformation across the globe, and it's mostly due to the advent of battery-powered technology. All of a sudden, biking is no longer limited to small kids, outdoor enthusiasts, and competitive racers. It's been democratized!

The convenience of a bike was never a diminished attribute. We just failed to acknowledge it. Straddling a bike, strapping on a helmet, and gliding down a hill is one of the more freeing feelings an adult can have at the cost of little effort. Which leads me to efficiency. I've had many a moment of chagrin in Portland, waiting in a line of backed-up automobiles to progress through a four-way intersection, to see one of my neighbors, or three, glide past on their bikes and on toward their destination, skirting the car conga line without a whim or care. I'd sit there looking on and wonder to myself, *Why aren't I smart enough to do what they're doing?*

When I was living in Amsterdam, I biked. I biked everywhere and to everything. On an apartment-hunting trip a few months before we officially moved to Europe, my husband and I were walking around the city trying to get a feel for the neighborhoods and where we wanted to reside. We would stop and ask Dutch men and women how far a certain location or museum was from where we were standing, and they'd kindly quote a time estimate for reaching our destination of choice. We never could understand why it always took us double or triple the time to get there from the time quoted. After we bought bikes, we understood. Everything in Amsterdam is quoted in bike time. And without fail, biking between any two locations was the fastest, most efficient mode of transport in the city. Biking beat driving, walking, taking the tram, and definitely the subway any time, any day of the week.

With the advent of ebikes, all of our horizons have expanded, and beautifully so. Biking is no longer an activity just for the physically fit. Biking is not just for individuals who live on flat terrain. Biking is not just for urban dwellers with short work commutes.

Biking is for the old, the young, and all those in between. Biking is for urban, suburban, and rural living. Ebikes convert biking from a perceived obstacle—in terms of convenience, comfort, and efficiency—to an opportunity. Thus, biking becomes an exercise in choice: to choose the outdoors and fresh air, to choose to commune with nature, and to choose physical activity and health. Cycling, whether on a standard or electric-powered ebike, emits zero carbon and leaves no impact on the earth.

What else can I tease you with? Biking is awesome. And it's particularly good for you physically, emotionally, and psychologically.

It's physical exercise that is nonstrenuous and low impact. The act of biking is a proven stress reliever and supports weight loss. I mean, if you could be the great Wizard of Oz pulling levers to create magic, you would achieve perfection by making a bike appear.

Public versus Private

I'm an urban gal. For much of my adult life, taking public transportation has been not only very accessible but also an integral lever I employed to get me to where I needed to go on a daily basis. I've lived in almost all of the major East Coast cities: Philadelphia, New York City, Boston, and Washington, DC. Throw in several extended living stints in Munich and Amsterdam and my current home of Portland, Oregon, and I've got the urban thing well under my ample knowledge belt. Commuting in every city is different, of course. In DC, I rode the subway system. In Philly, I walked, biked, and hopped on the city's SEPTA, the regional commuter rail, to visit my aunt Rosemary, who lived a block off the R5 line, snag a homemade meal, and wash my laundry for free. In NYC, it was walking and riding the subhuman (as my aunt loved to call it), the city's comprehensive subway system. I scrapped the car I had bought in my senior year of college and lived car-free for ten delicious years. In Boston, I walked and loved hopping on the MBTA subway system that ran cars above and below ground.

I know public transit systems, and I appreciate the ones that make your life easier and not more complicated. Philadelphia's? Eh, not so great, and the process of finding a stop took longer than just walking to where I needed to be. DC's is a hub-and-spoke system. It worked well when my to-and-from destinations were found on the ring of the wheel. Otherwise, traveling from one spoke to the other was frightfully drawn out. Portland is the only city in the US I have found is better designed for biking than using public transportation. I do admire the fairly young streetcar system that runs through and links four of the city's five downtown quadrants (yes, you read that right) to make the city more accessible, with an eye toward promoting social equity, affordable mobility, and economic vibrancy.

How we commute and get ourselves around taking care of life's many necessities is important. It's deadly important if how we do that is through the use of a combustion-engine automobile. Deadly, in that all that combusted gas is terrible for the earth, polluting our air, and making our lungs and bodies sick.

Here is another relevant question: Can our road infrastructure sustain all our cars today, let alone all the possible cars that will be on the roads, tomorrow? High rates of population growth (concentrated in cities) are placing increasing burdens on existing road infrastructure already overtaxed and in need of wholesale repair. In the US, the federal government's highway system has been chronically underfunded, requiring $836 billion in highway and bridge funding. The American Society of Civil Engineers estimates that a third of all urban roads in the US are in poor condition.[4] All told, Americans spend nearly 7 billion hours in delayed traffic, wasting 3 billion gallons of fuel while idling: a cost of $160 billion in lost time and wasted fuel, and another $112 billion in auto repair costs.[5] That is a lot of waste in time, money, and gas. Why not consider an alternative to car travel?

RENEE FRY

Cost and mental ease factors
of public transportation

RENEE FRY is an entrepreneur and adjunct professor who lives outside of Boston in Quincy, Massachusetts, with her husband and ten-year-old son. She's a registered Republican but votes Independent. Her house resides on the one-square-mile peninsula of Houghs Neck. It is 1,500 square feet and was built in 1920. She commutes twice a week into Cambridge, where she teaches, which is a twenty-seven-mile one-way ride from her home.

Renee knows she's lucky. Boston and its surrounding suburbs have an easily accessible and efficient public transportation system known as the "T" for short. She's very cognizant of the fact that most of her personal carbon footprint comes from using a combustion-engine car, which she owns. So, she finds ways to use her vehicle as little as possible.

Renee shares carpooling duties with her neighbors to cut down on single-passenger car use when driving a group of children the twelve-mile round trip to their elementary school. Where she feels she makes the biggest impact is by using Boston's subway system into Cambridge and back. Renee rattles off the many benefits from using public transportation twice a week:

- Avoiding car maintenance and gas costs

- Bypassing Boston's "horrendous" commuting traffic

- Saving $100 in parking costs each week, a net $5,000 in total (versus $25 per week and $1,250 in total spent purchasing round-trip train tickets)

Renee knows small sustainability actions are meaningful. Individual actions add up to make a big impact on mitigating climate change.

Sustainable Transportation Choices

For the Penny-Wiser	• Telecommute for work. • Use public transport for weekend outings.
For the Be-Bester	• Walk to complete your errands. • Bike with your kids to school.
For the Bridge Builder	• Organize a carpool to drive kids to and from school. • Take vacation road trips instead of long-haul holiday flights.
For the Nature Lover	• Lease or buy an EV or hybrid • Walk to grab lunch and/or a midday coffee.

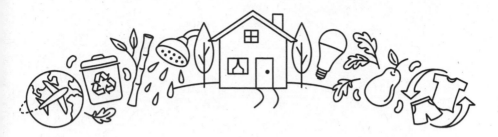

8

....

Energy

Like every other
viable environmental
policy, the search
for clean energy
begins at home.

ROGER SCRUTON

WHEN YOU walk into your home, you expect the lights to turn on with a flip of a switch or a turn of a knob. When you plug a cord into an outlet to install your TV, printer, and computer, you expect them to receive power and work just as they should, allowing you to enjoy on-demand shows, print recipes, and communicate with friends via social media. With that thermometer contraption on various walls of your house, you expect "ON" means air will flow to either heat or cool your home at whatever temperature you deem appropriate. These things are a given, right? Electricity, central heat, and air conditioning are a fundamental part of your human existence. At least here in the US and other developed countries and regions of the world. Unless high winds or heavy snowstorms knock out your power, you don't enter your home in the evening and light candles or make a fire to illuminate a room. You flick a switch and electricity—energy—is right there.

All that the above takes is a quick call to your local utility company to tell them to turn on the energy to your house or apartment. After that, you receive a monthly bill for energy use. Simple. But it's not. Most energy that has electrified and warmed our homes over the last one-hundred-plus years has been mined from the earth's interior. Those energy sources are oil, gas, and coal. Coal is dark, dirty, energy-packed rock mined from the depths of the planet. Many humans have lost their lives, livelihoods, and health from mining coal. If miners don't contract black lung disease, there's always the threat of a collapsed mine entrapping and often killing them. Coal mining is an extractive process that denudes the earth of soils and requires enormous amounts of water for processing, leaving behind contaminated surface water and groundwater aquifers laced with harmful chemicals such as lead, arsenic, and cadmium. It's a good energy source for heating but really awful for people to breathe and terrible for the earth when burned, releasing chemicals and trapping carbon dioxide in the atmosphere.

Oil is slick, dark, gooey, and rather to be avoided from a human-touch standpoint. It's also rich in energy. Oil has to be drilled—on land; out at sea—and forced from the earth's core. It's noxious by itself, but chemicals also have to be used to refine and convert it to the gasoline we pump into our cars and trucks. Those chemicals and the vapors from the refining process are, again—I hate to repeat myself, but I'm trying to make a point here—bad for the air we breathe and the health of the individuals who work in this industry. Tar, fumes, and chemical-laced water runoff from oil refineries are toxic to humans, wildlife, and marine life. Water pollution from spills and leaks is devastating, decimating marine species and the livelihoods of individuals that make a living from the water. Air pollution is an ever-present reality.

Natural gas, particularly of the fracking kind that is predominant here in America, is found trapped in air pockets between sedimentary rock and either piped or blasted out. Fracking is immensely costly, environmentally damaging, and insidious: the highly pressurized hydraulics used to crack rock and release natural gas from deep within the earth's rock layers can cause earthquakes. In addition, a huge amount of water, chemicals, and sand are used to force out fracked gas from these enclosed rock pockets. Do you want the bad news or the bad news on natural gas? The first bad is that all that water and chemical use contaminates our groundwater aquifers—think of these as huge, pristine, underground freshwater lakes—as well as our surface water bodies. We pay for this "natural" energy source with wrecked water. Contamination of our aquifers could easily destroy the best sources of fresh water humans need for survival. And, of course, like the other two fossil fuel energy sources, the burning of natural gas contributes mightily to increasing air temperatures that exacerbate our climate change problem. That's the second bad.

These energy sources—coal, oil, and natural gas—have been the mighty three for a long time. And in the near past, if you had called your utility, these would have been the default energy options provided to you to heat, cool, and electrify your home.

They are not worth it anymore. And, you have many options—increasingly so—to opt out of fossil fuels and opt in to sourcing, supporting, and growing the production of renewable energy sources that are

- not detrimental to your health;
- not sticky;
- not smelly;
- not noxious;
- not emissions-producing;
- not tearing up the earth to be extracted; and
- not polluting our freshwater supplies.

The sun shines and we transform its energy (solar). The water moves and we harness its energy (hydro). The wind whips and we convert its energy (wind). The oceans flow and we capture that energy (tidal). The earth holds a steady temperature and we harness that energy (geothermal).

Our choice of energy is stark. Do we continue to mine and burn noxious hydrocarbons to ensure that we are comfortable, lighted, and safe in our homes, or do we tap a vast system of energy sources that feel good, are good, and equally serve our basic needs of comfort and ease of use? My bet is on the latter.

We have set up a perverse system across the globe to use energy sources that have far worse side effects than the problems they seek to solve. We need energy to light our homes and businesses. We need energy to heat and cool our houses and buildings. We need energy to heat our water. And we need energy to propel our transportation systems, including our cars, trucks, trains, buses, and airplanes.

Wood has been a source of energy since the days of the cavemen. Then came coal, a black rock burned for its heat intensity. Coal's been around a long time. It's been traced back 3,500 years in China as a heat source. Petroleum, better known as oil and the refined gas that fills our gas tanks, was discovered in the late 1800s in America and became a boom industry in Texas and Oklahoma at the turn of the century. Natural gas brings up the rear in fossil fuel sources. Discovered in the mid-1950s in the US, it became one of the pillars of America's national energy security during the Nixon years, was supported by deregulated markets in the mid-1980s under the Reagan administration, and exploded as one of the primary and relatively inexpensive sources of energy in the US beginning in the mid-1990s. We should give a nod to nuclear power, given that the first atomic bomb was detonated in the summer of 1945 at Los Alamos, New Mexico, giving rise to the proliferation of nuclear weapons and their by-product, nuclear-powered energy plants. The first nuclear power plant became operational in America in 1958.

The two outliers in these energy sources are wood and nuclear power. Wood is technically a renewable resource because it comes from trees, and trees can be replanted by humans easily and successfully. I'll talk about nuclear power in a moment.

The need for energy is a very human condition. We seek light in the dark, warmth from the cold, and coolness from the heat. As societies have modernized and individuals seek comforts beyond their immediate needs, energy sources provide for our needs but also fuel our wants and desires for entertainment, electronic gadgets, travel, and productivity gains. This is natural. Our energy cravings from fossil fuels have detrimental side effects. And they've been accumulating for hundreds of years. We've known acutely about those ill effects for at least the last fifty years. The problem is Big Oil and the beneficiaries of their largess—the government, politicians, and industry lobbyists—want to keep us hooked on fossil fuel energy. Big Oil companies are making a killing in profits. So what if our water, land, and air is polluted in the process of mining these energy sources? Why should they care if the direct by-product of burning fossil fuels is the driving force of our climate crisis? Money, money, money! Give me the money!

You should care.

Nuclear
· · · · · · · · ·

And now a short discussion on nuclear power energy. Yes, the energy generated from nuclear power plants is emissions-free. The country of France is mostly (seventy-five percent) powered by clean nuclear energy. That's how it is able to achieve its low average per capita carbon emissions footprint of 4.6 metric tons. ·

Now, the actual construction of nuclear reactors is material-intensive and quite expensive, with an average price tag to operationalize a plant costing in the billions of dollars. And carbon-intensive.

My beef is with the radioactive waste nuclear power plants generate. Spent nuclear fuel rods, or the waste from the energy generated from the plant, must sit in pools of water; big pools of water to cool the rods down sufficiently to transfer them to a longer-term containment solution. If water levels are not sufficiently maintained or are disrupted by a natural disaster, the rods can heat up and cause a nuclear explosion with serious consequences to human and environmental health. We know how deadly those can be. Think Chernobyl, a nuclear reactor meltdown resulting in part from human error, or, more recently in 2011, the Fukushima Daiichi Nuclear Power Plant meltdown triggered by an offshore tsunami.

Spent radioactive fuel rods can also be buried, placed in canisters that are enclosed in tunnels sealed with rocks and clay.[1] Call it "deep" burial. Every year, two thousand metric tons of spent fuel rods need to be managed: soaked in water pools for three to ten years and then transported to underground storage casks to effectively decompress in order to become non-lethal to living organisms. Since the first nuclear reactor plant was operationalized in the 1950s, some eighty-five thousand metric tons of nuclear waste has been generated. Fifty-five nuclear power plants remain active in the US as of 2021.[2]

Waste keeps accumulating. There exists no permanent storage facility for spent rods today. And unlike France, the US recycles none of its nuclear material fuel, soaking and burying it instead. That waste will be radioactive—deadly to humans and every other living organism—for some 250,000 years.[3]

So, even though all the nuclear waste arguably fits well within the size of one football field, it exists and keeps on becoming more of a problem that has yet to be solved. I worry about our water resources being allocated to waste that requires diligence and oversight over a scale of decades, if not centuries. Humans, let alone politicians, have a hard time planning ahead four decades, let alone 2,500 centuries. I am concerned about accidental contamination of our soils and groundwater aquifers.

I ask you: Why would we knowingly continue to rely on this source of energy when the by-products of its use have a small but acute potential of destroying that which we rely on to nourish us and keep us healthy and alive?

There is a better way. We know that way: renewables.

Centralized versus Distributed

For almost 140 years, Americans have taken for granted that their energy, their electricity, came from a "utility," a public entity that generated and distributed energy to our homes and businesses. If we moved to a new state, we'd look up who our state or regional utility was and sign up to have them deliver power to our new home. Our options were minimal to none. We called one provider to flick our switch "on" and waited (impatiently) for the energy to flow. Most utilities in the US are publicly traded, although here in the Pacific Northwest, we have federally owned and managed utilities. Throughout this first century and a half, energy generation and distribution was a nationally regulated market that was centrally managed. The naughts brought deregulation to the energy markets. And with it came the rise of renewable energy: energy created through natural systems and renewable energy sources.

Renewables are diversified energy sources. They don't come from one power plant. Think about it: sun is dispersed energy. We can capture it on the sides of walls, on rooftops, via solar farms across swaths of open land, and from movable panels. Wind is also dispersed energy. By its very nature, it moves and flows. It's windier on tops of hills without the benefit of tree coverage than thick in a forest surrounded by thirty-foot trees. The same goes for hydropower, which is electricity generated from the flow and movement of water, mainly through dams. There are other forms of renewable energies, such as geothermal (heat sourced from the earth's interior), tidal, and biomass (heat generated from wood, plants, and biowaste). Because these renewable energy sources come from different regions, methods, and mechanisms, these types of energy are in *distributed* form.

Distributed also means that energy sources can serve and support more localized groups of buildings or individuals. Solar panels on a home can serve one family. A solar-powered microgrid can serve a small community. Biomass energy can run a co-packing factory that serves five businesses.

Renewable energy is diversified—it comes in many forms—and works best in a distributed way—serving the needs of one to many. Renewable energy can be stand-alone, sourced and used on its own, or it can be connected to a utility. When it is connected, it can "feed" the centralized grid—provide extra energy to the grid—or be supported by it, gaining continuity of energy when the source of renewable energy is not readily available, say when a bad nor'easter blows in and sits above your city for five days longer than expected, blocking out the sun.

Because distributed energy can be localized, it is an option for homeowners looking to ensure they are using renewable energy at home. Homeowners have three main distributed energy systems to consider when deciding to go renewable:

- Solar photovoltaic (PV): Think solar panels on your roof.

- Solar thermal: This is a newer type of technology (although quite prevalent in Europe) that uses the sun's energy to heat a substance (e.g., water, oil, air) to effectively and efficiently heat rooms in a home.

- Geothermal loop: Also called a geothermal heat pump or ground-source heat pump, it is an underground system of pipes that harnesses the constant temperature of the earth (54°F) by moving fluid through the system to heat and cool your home and water.

Installing a renewable energy (RE) system on your home or property most definitely helps to decrease your "operating" cost of living. That said, that is not the typical reason individuals install solar panels or geothermal loops. Most who decide to make a financial investment in solar or geothermal systems are declaring in a definitive way that sourcing RE is good for the planet's health and is a sustainable source of energy that stops their consumption of carbon-emitting fossil fuels. It's an outward statement of an internal ethos: I care about Earth and its ability to sustain life.

We need both forms of energy, centralized and distributed. Both energy systems are made more durable and resilient by the advantages and capabilities each system provides. Both become more sustainable as they work together to build each other's "green" capacity: onboarding higher percentages of renewable energy sources to support the movement toward renewables, withdrawing our dependency on fossil fuels, and ensuring that demand peaks and energy intermittencies are smoothed.

Energy Storage

What gal doesn't like a little extra storage? Look over here. I'm raising my hand, big-time! Storage: you have it because you come to realize you need it.

So it is with renewable energy. Storing distributed—renewable—energy allows us to spread its use over the day and night hours and on sunny, rainy, or cloudy days. Renewable energy storage makes energy available to us when and where we need it so the light goes on when we flick a room switch, our smartphones get charged when we plug them in, the water runs hot on frigid weekday mornings, and the heat and air conditioning keep us perfectly content as we go about our days, weeks, and months of living, loving, and relaxing at home.

The sun's rays are intermittent. The sun doesn't reliably shine every day, twenty-four hours a day. Especially in particular parts of the world. In Amsterdam, I felt sun deprived; it rained so much. The same is true of wind. Some parts of the world are windy. Chicago in the winter comes to mind. So does any mountainous region of the US, whether that be the White Mountains in New Hampshire or Government Camp at the base of Mount Hood in Oregon. But other places, not so much.

Intermittency is when the sun stops shining, the wind stops blowing, the water stops flowing, or factory workers go home for the night and stop processing plant compost for energy.

Renewable energy is cool. It's the future. It can provide us with all the energy we need. But we need to capture it—store it—during times when it's really sunny and windy so it's available to use when it's cloudy, rainy, or calm outside. Storage helps spread energy abundance during times when it is (naturally) lacking.

Storage is there when we anticipate the expected. Like the solar-powered generator installed by the owners of the Glen Ellen home in Sonoma, California, where my family and I decamped to during the summer of 2020. The home was on the top of a hill, basking in sun most days and months. The owners knew that rolling blackouts by the state utility PG&E were becoming a common annual occurrence during the late summer and early fall months, to prevent fires from starting. The generator was installed to ensure that if a planned (or unplanned) blackout occurred, its residents would still have access to electricity, hot water, and a working stove.

Storage. It comes in handy. It helps us optimize our lives. In this case, it organizes our energy systems so we expect continuity while building resilience and embracing sustainability. Go renewables!

MELODY JONES

The Powerwall

MELODY JONES is a single, early-fifties professional who resides in Sausalito, California. She rents a second-floor in-law suite from her landlord, an East Coast transplant. In his six years of owning property in California, Melody's landlord has experienced the growing wildfires in the region and has been directly impacted by the unplanned rolling blackouts instituted by the embattled California utility provider, PG&E. Just before the summer of 2019, he installed a Powerwall. The Powerwall is manufactured by the electric vehicle manufacturer Tesla and is a rechargeable lithium-ion battery storage device. It is solar powered and for home use.

When I called Melody in mid-summer 2019 to ask how she was being affected by the weeks-long rolling blackout that was crippling the economic productivity of San Francisco and its surrounding neighborhoods, throwing communities and homes into darkness for much of the working daylight hours, she was unperturbed. She told me that her landlord had anticipated the rolling blackouts and installed a Powerwall to ensure that the duplex had continuity of electricity. And it had done its job well. She was unaffected by the blackouts and could work and use electricity for her personal and professional needs without worry. Melody said that the Powerwall was a godsend, really, since it meant she did not have to worry or plan alternative means for living and working during a very disruptive time.

Sustainable Energy Choices

For the Penny-Wiser	• Purchase high-efficiency dish and clothing washers and dryer. • Use only the cold-water/eco setting on dish and clothing washers.
For the Be-Bester	• Replace gas range with electric (induction) option. • Buy monthly, quarterly, or annual carbon offsets for personal carbon emissions.
For the Bridge Builder	• Install a PV solar panel system to heat the home and water. • Source renewable energy from a local utility or retail energy supplier.
For the Nature Lover	• Install a geothermal system to supply electricity for the home. • Cool the home using passive air conditioning strategies (e.g., shades drawn in day, windows open at night).

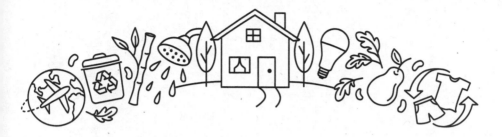

9

....

Home and Property

Have nothing in
your houses that you
do not know to
be useful or believe
to be beautiful.

WILLIAM MORRIS

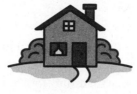

WILLIAM RANDOLPH HEARST, the larger-than-life newspaper man, broke ground in 1919 on his over-the-top vision of a home and playground for him and his many prestigious friends on what was pristine coastal and cattle-ranching land. For nearly thirty years, he worked alongside Julia Morgan, the respected architect, to not quite complete the building of a monolithic series of structures to house mostly two people, Hearst and his mistress, the Hollywood actress Marion Davies. The Spanish-style castle, with many overt references to European empires and mythology, is one giant homage to wealth, excess, and—let's be real—ego. At Hearst Castle, now a museum, one can find four structures, encompassing over eighty thousand square feet in its footprint, and two gargantuan pools, aptly named Neptune and Roman. In the main living quarters, Casa Grande, Hearst commissioned Morgan to build a 68,000-square-foot home that included thirty-eight bedrooms, forty-two bathrooms, and fourteen sitting rooms! Compare that to the average US home today, clocking in at 2,687 square feet.[1]

The planning and construction of the Hearst home bankrupted him many millions over. And to what end? Hearst Castle reflects a different life, time, and era; one that held no notion of what sustainability is and, from a material standpoint, held a low value of it.

The Case for Small
· ·

Big homes demand lots of materials to build them. Most of those materials are brand-new, virgin-sourced, hot off the manufacturing floor. And by virgin, I mean materials sourced for the very first time, including wood from trees and aluminum, steel, and plastic from mined oil and natural gas. Big homes require a large land footprint in square footage and acres, land that once held trees, grass, and topsoil. These acted like living sponges to soak up carbon dioxide in the air and naturally and beautifully absorb rain- and storm-water, which they deposited like a gift to our underground reservoir pools—groundwater aquifers—to clean and purify the fresh water on which all life depends. The building footprints of homes seal away—and steal—the earth's ability to make this even exchange, and instead hardens and makes impenetrable the land on which a home sits. Greenfields make way for cement fields.

It reminds me of a trip I made to the Mütter Museum in Philadelphia, when I was studying for my master's in business administration at the University of Pennsylvania. The Mütter Museum is a repository of medical history, both of the ordinary and the bizarre. It was there that I looked upon the skeletal histories of individuals who were diagnosed with fibrodysplasia ossificans progressiva, also known as Münchmeyer disease. Münchmeyer disease is an extremely rare disorder that transforms a person's connective tissues—muscle, tendons, and ligaments—into bone. Individuals with this disorder become paralyzed and incapacitated as their bodies slowly but steadily ossify. The construction of homes has a similar effect on the planet: calcifying the place where they sit.

Big homes require more energy to heat and cool themselves. And big homes, by necessity, require things to fill them up and make them homey, cozy, comfortable, and beautiful.

Millennials have embraced a smart way of living large: occupying and buying smaller homes with a tighter footprint that are efficient, require less energy and material inputs, and maximally serve their lifestyle needs. Millennial families are smaller, averaging fewer than three people per home. They work hard for their money, which is spread thinner than that of previous generations, and seek to live simply and well, balancing a home that is comfortable, environmentally friendly, and cost-efficient to heat, cool, and maintain. Their emphasis is on an experiential life that marries a love of the outdoors and the amenities it provides with the safety, security, and convenience of a home with a light impact on the world.

The financial affordability and significant savings that can be realized by living small extends to college students, empty nesters, and elderly people, disparate populations that have a common goal: to unburden themselves of the work, care, and constant upkeep large homes require.[2] We are in a boom of building tiny-home communities across the US and in urban areas, where houses can range from sixty to five hundred square feet in size. Some eighteen states and growing have passed legislation allowing for accessory dwelling units (ADUs) to be built on existing private home properties. These units can provide a larger footprint, between two hundred and eight hundred square feet, to occupants, but there is minimal care required because the necessities of living have been stripped down to the bare essentials.

You may not be a millennial, an empty nester, or retired. You may be like me, a medium-aged working woman and wife raising two young children. Life is busy, complicated, challenging, and very nearly requiring a level of sophisticated multitasking that makes you exhausted just thinking about it. Smaller homes, in a size that is comfortable and accommodating, efficient and affordable, welcoming and endearing, are arguably what we may be craving during these increasingly uncertain times. Consider, then, that bigger may not be better, medium may be just right for now, and smaller a reachable perfection as our lives evolve and demand more to be lived and less to be maintained.

Choosing Urban over Suburban
· ·

I grew up in the truly sleepy town of Vienna, Virginia, the total size of which spanned a three-by-three-mile radius. House doors were left open and ignition keys left in unlocked, parked cars during the day. Kids ran the neighborhoods, with neighbors watching on and over. The hottest spot in town on a weekend night was the McDonald's on Maple Avenue, Vienna's main central street.

Vienna resides just seventeen miles south of Washington, DC, and is a suburban haven nearly subsumed these days by the bustling and growing city seat of our federal government. I left for college life in rural New Hampshire and landed in Boston upon graduation. And urban I have remained since. Urban is the only life for me.

I'm not alone, it turns out. Urban cities are growing more popular and populous by the day. Some eighty-three percent of the total population in the US lives in urban areas, nearly a twenty percent increase from 1950 numbers. Within thirty years, come the year 2050, an additional seven percent of the US population will be urban residents.[3] People are choosing to live closer together, at higher density levels than at any time during our collective history. Let's look at this phenomenon with a sustainability lens.

Let's go back to my little town of Vienna. It's grown up in the thirty years since I left it, but the way in which its residents get around has not. Most people live in single-family homes or small-rise condominiums. Typical lots are a quarter of an acre in size. Lawns are well manicured, and private property boundaries are well demarcated with "white" picket-fencing. Most everyone has to drive to the local grocery store, pharmacy, or restaurant. Owning a vehicle is a necessity. If you start on one side of the town and drive to the other, Vienna provides a microcosm of other suburban town experiences: fast-food restaurants, franchise retailers, and national service chains populate and repeat themselves across the landscape—the strip-malling of America. We seek to provide convenience through replication, redundancy, and a leveling-down of unique experience. I call it the ditto effect of suburban life: a déjà vu experience that is familiar in its uniformity yet disheartening in its repetition.

In city life, there is proximity, vibrancy, and immediacy.

Take the city of Amsterdam, the international metropolis of the Netherlands, considered one of the world's most sustainable cities. Bikes are king there. A biker can report to police officers absent-minded or malignant car drivers that cause them perceived (or real) harm by obstructing passageways on the vast network of dedicated biking lanes that crisscross the city. Bikers have right of way at four-way intersections. Cars must look out for bikers before they park and pull out of parking spaces. Lovers hold hands down a street as they ride along on their mutual bikes. Date nights are performed by riding a bike from home to a restaurant and jazz club and back. Moms and dads ride bikes everywhere with their little kids, starting as young as six months, when infants have the ability to hold the weight of their own heads. The frequent sightings tug at your heart strings: bike seats in front with Plexiglas windows protecting babes from outdoor elements. Older kids sit behind their parents, some with arms around their waists. Multiple children will be in tented Bakfiets, sturdy wood or Plexiglas carriages hitched to the front of a bike, that adeptly weave and poke their way through streets to their preferred destination.

Proximity

During my four years living in Amsterdam, driving a car was an afterthought, equally burdensome and unnecessary to daily life. The street on which my second-story apartment resided was Willemsparkweg, where the 2 and 5 tramlines that lead from Centraal Station to the outskirts of the metropolitan area offered stops every five blocks or so. I lived three blocks from the entrance to Vondelpark, the well-known "central park" of the city, although that's a misnomer, given the pure abundance of green space found there. Residents moved equally by bike, tram, and train for work, pleasure, and daily routine. Distances from here to there were quoted in bike times: ten minutes from Vondelpark to the Jordaan, fifteen minutes to Amsterdam Centraal Station, and five to the Dam. In fact, there's no location in the city of Amsterdam that takes longer than fifteen or twenty minutes to get to from any other point.

My grocery stores were either Organic or Albert Heijn (AH), located one and a half and four blocks, respectively, from my apartment. So too, the wine shop, eye shop, furniture shop, clothing stores, pharmacy, hardware store, and a gaggle of various restaurants: all were within a five-block radius of me. And that's the point: living life and conducting its mundane yet necessary tasks were in foot-shot of my home. Most every shop except the national grocery store, AH, was independently owned. I knew, unequivocally, that my euros spent supported a collective of entrepreneurs relying and thriving on a local community. The level of proximity for living a good life on foot or by bike cannot be denied.

Immediacy

The city of New York is such a unique place to live. When I first moved there in 2000, post-graduate school and so cash poor I had to ask for a loan from my new employer, Time Inc., in order to rent a U-Haul to move my meager possessions into a friend's apartment, I was struck by an overwhelming sense of sadness that emanated from Manhattanites, who seemed to scurry back and forth like roly-polies from an uplifted forest rock, without pausing or consideration for the moments that were ticking by in their lives. My affinity to NYC in those early days wavered between love and hate. Acceptance came in waves. I resided downtown in Chelsea, and I came to know, love, and frequent my favorite joints in the neighborhood: the long-gone LGBTQ+-friendly coffee house, The Big Cup; the corner French bistro, Le Grainne Cafe; my go-to authentic Italian restaurant, Le Zie; and the then newish Chelsea Market, an urban food, beverage, and dining bazaar. People knew me at these places. A market milk entrepreneur would engage me in conversation every time I entered his shop. He knew my favorite ice cream shake. The French bistro would see me and call out, "You want your ratatouille crepe?" and I nodded yes. In a city of

8 million, where I could be entirely anonymous on the city streets or riding the hot, crowded underground labyrinth of New York City's subway system, bonds of unspoken friendship and intimacy were forged between independent producers and urban consumers.

Vibrancy

My husband and I would coax each other when we lacked the energy to leave the den of our humble yet homey fourth-floor apartment in Manhattan with an often-used axiom, "Let's just get our feet on the street and we'll be happy we did." Yes, NYC can be a daunting place, with trash bags piled wall high on pickup day, the waft of urine down the long city blocks, and the sheer aggressiveness of its citizens as they make their way to destinations near, far, and unknown. But just the same, the city has life and breathes excitement and energy into the individuals who live there. NYC offers a world of opportunity to experience culture and the arts at such a breadth and depth, it's hard to limit yourself to one choice daily.

The Joyce Theater, a fewer-than-five-hundred-seat dance performance venue, was my first of many forays experiencing modern dance at an elite level. I feasted on off-off-Broadway theater, where the venues were small, discreet, and often near-hidden, and that put on one- and two-person productions that both riveted and satisfied me. I sought out the speakeasies, those old-time secret drinking haunts that still exist but are no longer verboten, to experience in some small way what form "having some fun" took during Prohibition. I reveled in late-night jam sessions at some of the city's most notorious and well-known jazz clubs. And ah, the delights of Lincoln Center; that glorious front of imposing buildings beckoned me to experience classical operas and circus performances in equal measure. These moments of cultural connection made me feel truly a part of the city, its true beating heart these diverse communities vibrant and alive. Wherever you are, just getting your feet on the street connects you to your community intimately and in real time.

DURING THE 2020 doldrums, cities emptied out as their residents scattered to less populated, less dense regions, a chance to get away and be free of heavy burdens literally hanging in the air. Cities became quieter. Some experienced cleaner air. Life in some sense condensed to a simpler cadence for those who stayed: communing on the open streets, in the expansive parks, and with each other, exercising abundant care. The vibrancy, immediacy, and proximity of urban living cannot be denied for long. Slowly, inevitably, and with a sense of destiny, city life will be reborn, reinvented, and renewed, and those who return to live alongside their fellow neighbors reinvigorated by all the chaos, electric energy, and "madding" crowds urbanites love to hate and hate to miss.

City life provides that density and intensity of experience. Diversity abounds. Tensions flare, yes, but one knows that to get along we must sometimes accept, sometimes endure, and always consider others with care. Crowded urban living disallows seated dinner parties in expansive homes. But it does provide access to an extraordinary amount of culture, simple touchpoints, and individuals to connect and thrive through curiosity, creativity, and kindness. Urban life connects us to humanity so intimately that we cannot help to see ourselves in the lives and plights of others. Because we cannot avoid our urban fellow "man," equally alike and dissimilar to ourselves, there is a process that unfolds in parallel as life marches forward: of both seeking to understand and accepting others for who they are. It's a beautiful thing, and an experience I value.

Cities will continue to remain beacons of sustainable living, where the very nature of urbanism means growing housing options for a diverse set of socioeconomic communities, denser housing that accommodates better living, and commuting options for city dwellers, including accessible walking paths and pedestrian-only zones, biking paths that replace car lanes, and multitudes of mixed-use retail neighborhoods that offer a richness of options for eating, drinking, playing, and convening with a diverse community of like-minded individuals.

Old and Renewed:
The Value of Place, History, and Story
· ·

My jaunts down to Miami Beach during my twenties, when I felt
like a jetsetter, dating a French man from Paris, no less, were dis-
orienting. I was living in the South End of Boston proper, a former
strip of marsh land filled in by municipal planners to increase
the residential space of the city. The neighborhood historically
attracted African American homeowners and gay tenants shut
out of the upper-middle-class and predominantly white Back Bay
neighborhood. The South End was designed by Charles Bulfinch,
a renowned architect, back in the 1850s. He created wide, tree-
lined streets that scattered small green parks with fountains as
centerpieces among stately rows of single-family brick townhouses
accented with iron railings and small front garden plots, which
made the neighborhood visually appealing and historically and
architecturally significant.

Miami Beach was another world entirely. Nearly every structure was stucco and a variation on a pink, bumblebee-yellow, and
baby-blue theme. With the exception of the rundown Art Deco
buildings that line Ocean Drive, the main nightlife strip of Miami
Beach, most buildings found in the city were low-slung, newly built
structures that lacked any discernible tie to historical influence. I
had the distinct impression that once these somewhat amorphous
buildings began to show their wear, they were simply torn down
to make way for the new. I lacked a point of reference: What was
historical and why? What was the essence of this city, or was rein-
vention its heart and soul?

This story comes around to be punctuated by my years living
in Amsterdam and New York City. In Manhattan and the other
boroughs of New York City spanning a hundred-year timeframe
starting in 1840, the construction of multilevel mixed-use commercial buildings with storefronts and ornamental features using
a "revolutionary" material—cast iron—became de rigueur. A New
Yorker and self-taught architect and engineer, James Bogardus,

began building the city using cast iron as his muse, proselytizing, rightly, the material's superior attributes: strength, structural stability, durability, malleability, and fire-resistance, a particularly useful quality during the industrial age.[4] Today, developers wanting to build in areas designated a "historic district" in Manhattan are required by NYC's Landmarks Preservation Commission to preserve cast iron architectural elements and, increasingly, entire facades. Walking in the city, you can see razed buildings with their facades still standing, empty caverns with their pretty faces readying for a makeover. It is at once humbling and remarkable: the value the city places on historical preservation and the revitalization of America's particular class of dinosaurs that will remain to continue telling their story.

The city of Amsterdam and its architectural history go back far earlier than that of Manhattan, to the twelfth century. But as in NYC, the Industrial Revolution provided the impetus for "the city of canals" to grow its core beyond the Singelgracht, to build working and residential neighborhoods that are today designated prime city real estate. I lived in one of these tall, slim brick-facade buildings with massive windows on Willemsparkweg, in the neighborhood of Oud-Zuid, built during the industrial era between 1813 and the 1940s. The city of Amsterdam, just like Manhattan, has strict restoration and preservation regulations that building developers and landlords must abide by. In my second-story apartment, there were two "shower stalls" and one toilet closet. The original toilet "room" had once been a small balcony, renovated and enclosed to be incorporated into the house for hygienic use. In that small room, which housed a flushing toilet and sink, with no room to spare, was an immense stained glass window, part of the outer wall of the original building structure. It had been reinforced—protected—both internally and externally, with clear glass panels to ensure that nothing would happen to it. I found out through the landlord that the stained glass window could not be removed and must be left in its original place to ensure the historical integrity of the house; a beautiful yet awkwardly placed remnant of a long-ago era.

All this is to say, history and place matter. The old can be renewed again, with care and consideration. Bringing a wrecking ball to buildings abandoned or in various states of disrepair destroys our history as we know it or have yet to reveal. There is value in historical significance. Care and consideration of what has been and what can be are reconcilable goals. I understand that some of us value history and cherish the old, while others value the new and modern. Renewing existing structures bridges the divide between old and new and provides value to both sides and aesthetic mindsets.

I have a dear friend who bought a house in the Shepherd Park neighborhood of Washington, DC, back in the mid-naughts. It is located in the northern "point" of the district, just south of Silver Spring, Maryland, a historically diverse, tight-knit community. She bought a grand old house built in 1915. She's a gal who loves old things and big restoration projects. She quickly found out post-move that every single one of the house's windows had been caulked and silicone-sealed. Not a one could be opened in the sweltering months of late spring and summer. She set to meticulously unsealing each window and restoring them to their functional use.

I'm not like my friend, Melanie. I don't love the idea of spending years fixing up an old house while also living in a construction site. That said, I am a big believer in renewing old homes; honoring their bones and the place where they are sited and updating them with new amenities and construction materials that are highly insulating, high-efficiency, and well considered. The home I own was built in 1939. It sits on a hill overlooking downtown Portland. It was a historically spacious home, some 2,300 square feet, and was bought by a developer when its last owner moved into hospice. The developer approached the house's renovation with care. The bones of the home were kept: the rooms, the stairwells, and the fireplace. The foundation was reinforced up to code, so the house is not in jeopardy of sliding down the hill when/if the Cascadia subduction earthquake that is "overdue" hits the city. But the house was given enhanced features: new and highly efficient insulation, double-glazed low-E windows, a state-of-the-art tank-less water heater, and, on the house's backside, sliding windowed doors that provide an east-west air floor inside the house, cutting down on the need for mechanical ventilation during the spring to fall months. The building "envelope" did not increase from a land-use perspective, and no new impervious materials were added: the garage, sidewalk, and access to the street remained the same. Internal materials were reused, making salvage a priority over dem-olition and waste.

Living Small(er)

If you are looking to make a significant, long-term sustainability choice, consider living in a smaller space. This applies whether you rent or own your home. How should you measure "small"? As I mentioned, today's average new home size in the US is 2,687 square feet. How big is your current living space?

Now, that's the size of an average new home. A small home is considered to be approximately 1,660 square feet in total, which also happens to be the typical size of houses built in 1973. Compact is smaller than a small home. A compact home typically includes no more than 1,150 square feet. For comparison, the size of an aver-age two-bedroom apartment in New York City, San Francisco, and Chicago is 1,049 square feet, 1,013 square feet, and 996 square feet, respectively.[5] So, comparatively, compact living is also how many urban dwellers live. This type of smaller living is not only trending true in urban cities but is also more than accommodating for the size of a typical US household (2.53 occupants) as of 2020, which has been trending downward over the last half-century.[6]

JOHN TORGERSON

Living minimally

JOHN IS a man of deep conviction and quiet fortitude when it comes to living fully, presently, and sustainably. He and his wife, self-identified minimalists, reside in St. Paul, Minnesota, and are homeowners of a compact-sized house. Before pursuing a career as a real estate agent, where John actively advises individuals seeking home ownership to consider living small and to pursue rebuilding and reconstruction projects for older homes, he was a toolmaker who teamed with NASA to support projects such as its intrepid Martian rover, *Curiosity*, preparing it for its time on Mars.

John advocates publicly and professionally for others to live a sustainable life imbued with meaning, purpose, healthy choices, and conscious decision-making. John makes it clear that "the actions we take at home are the most meaningful." We have to stand up for what we believe, and living our belief system is the best example any of us can set for others.

John details the multitude of benefits he receives from his sustainable living choices. He is a homeowner of a "humble" place so that he can have full responsibility for the stewardship of the home and the property on which it sits. Because his home is small and "just meets his needs," his mortgage is manageable and will be paid off far more quickly than the typical thirty years. John states he spends far less on taxes, interest, and home maintenance. Given that he is a toolmaker and works on wood projects as a passion hobby, he notes that "he uses fewer materials on every [home] project." From a holistic life perspective, John uses less energy for heating and cooling his home and purchases fewer material things to decorate the living space, in John's words, "spending less on the things that don't matter."

It's notable that John also makes a point of saying that this "saved" money is not for saving's sake. In his mind, he and his wife reallocate these life savings to things and activities that provide "greater value to the quality of our lives," including purchasing better-made, longer-lasting clothing, making meals with local ingredients that are better for their bodies, and tending to their own urban garden to consume fresh produce that they share with their neighbors to build community. The sustainable decisions John makes support a life that is less stressful and low carbon-intensive.

John expresses a sentiment that harkens back to the first chapter of this book and the idea that sustainable living is an old idea with renewed relevance today. He says, "[Sustainability] is important to us. We see it as a responsibility as old as time, teachings of our ancestors that have been neglected."

Ownership and Remodeling

Many of us aspire to own our own home, considering it one of the best long-term investments we make in our life. If you are certain you want to be a homeowner, the next logical question to ask yourself is what kind of home you should buy: one newly constructed or existing? Newly constructed homes use new materials, many of which are derived from oil and gas, but they are usually more energy efficient than older homes. Existing homes tend to be older homes that can have inefficient heating, cooling, and insulation systems. In most cases, you'll seek to fix up or remodel an existing home to make it more contemporary, like new, or the embodiment of your personal design aesthetic. The same is true if you have lived in a home for quite a while and have decided, once and for all, that you are ready to upgrade the space to meet your current needs or desires.

If you want to upgrade an existing home, you have options involving varying degrees of sustainability.

- **Renovating a home:** an incremental process that is planned over a period of time, often accommodating the personal desires and financial constraints of a homeowner and involving little to no structural changes to an existing building, yet may entail significant material changes.

- **Remodeling a home:** a process whereby an existing building is updated or added onto, combining both new and old structures, but typically involving some form of demolition (or better, deconstruction, which involves dismantling a building piece by piece in an attempt to save and reuse as many of the building's components as possible[7]) to combine the old with the new as seamlessly as possible.

- **Rebuilding a home:** the "next level" of remodeling, involving taking an existing structure down to its bones to create something new but with thought and effort put toward trying to capture the embodied energy of an existing structure in some way. Capturing a house's embodied energy means respecting the viability and usefulness of existing materials by reusing them in a different way or recycling them so they are incorporated into new products (for example, using an old door to make a desk). A house rebuild requires a thoughtful pre-plan, third-party experts to help with the assessment and deconstruction of the home, and contractors knowledgeable in how to reuse and recycle all the salvageable components.

Home-building sustainability requires additional thought and planning and may demand greater upfront costs initially, but in the long run, much of the additional costs can be recouped in sales revenue, tax reductions, and city, state, or federal subsidies. Just as valuable are the mitigating impacts on resource use and landfill waste reduction, and the support provided by prolonging the life of valuable, recyclable home materials.

Property
· · · · · · · · · · ·

Chemical Use

One of the small but effective decisions we can make on sustainability is about the chemicals, fertilizers, and pesticides we use in and outside of our home maintaining our plants. If you are desperate to keep your flower garden or lawn looking tip-top, turn to the organic, natural-based fertilizers and pesticides the EPA suggests using. Any reputable nursery will be able to suggest organic alternatives. So too, big box home improvement stores stock organic lawn options. "Going organic" really involves a small shift in your buying decision-making, but it makes a huge difference in the amount of harmful, synthetic chemicals that enter waterways through stormwater runoff and seep into local soils and groundwater systems.

Synthetic fertilizers, herbicides, and pesticides acidify our waterways, zapping oxygen levels that fish and other marine organisms need to breathe, grow, and live. Perhaps alarmingly, what goes around, comes around. Harmful chemicals used on land plants find their way into the flesh of fish as well as aquatic insects that are part of the fish food chain. Many of these fish species we rely on for our own food intake. The circle of life is complete. We end up ingesting the exact chemicals we know to kill the weeds and pests we were so adamant to be rid of. This sounds gruesome, but it's more common than we realize. A study conducted by the city of Portland, Oregon, in 2007 found that wild salmon had dozens of synthetic chemicals in their systems.[8] *Scientific American* reported on another study in Indiana that found that "a variety of corn genetically engineered [GMO seeds] to produce the insecticide Bt is having toxic effects on non-target aquatic insects, including caddis flies, a major food source for fish and frogs."[9] The short of it is: it's not worth poisoning ourselves for a pretty, well-manicured lawn.

Lawn

We love our turf in America, but uniform green grass lawns are water hoggers and don't lend themselves well to promoting the local wildlife. Xeriscape lawns, however, flex some serious muscle in both the water-saving and biodiversity-promoting categories.

A xeriscaped landscape is a smart water-saving strategy that employs native and drought-resistant plants while avoiding lawn or turf planting. The plants typically picked for xeriscaping are water savers and native to your local region. If you live in a Western state that's typically dry year-round, exotic plants from South Africa, the Middle East, and Australia well adapted to long, dry seasons are a good choice.[10] For those living in the eastern parts of the US where the seasons are more differentiated—cold, wet, and snowy winters and warm, moist summers—picking native plants that are well adapted to local rainfall patterns is key.

Going "native" with your plant choices is a win for all: local pollinators are supported, local species are given food and shelter, and your plantings promote regional biodiversity.[11] So too, they require little to no fertilizers and minimal water maintenance, and they are more resistant to local pests and disease. Whether you're urban or rural, xeriscape lawns are a perfect choice.

Water Management

If you live in a city where there are large portions of land covered with impervious materials—homes, streets, driveways, sidewalks, commercial buildings—stormwater capture helps prevent water contaminants from everyday household items and activities (think gasoline, fertilizers, pesticides, paints, and chemicals) from polluting the municipal water system as well as local bodies of water, including lakes, rivers, creeks, and ponds. Because climate change is bringing more frequent and more violent weather events to land, managing the extreme influx of intense volumes of water onto your property is a smart adaptability measure that pays forward in more reliably clean, abundant water.

Cisterns and rain barrels help capture rainwater that falls on roofs and gutters. This helps prevent rainwater from washing over cemented surfaces or down steep hills to create floods, landslides, and river overflows. Underground cisterns, appropriately installed, allow you to capture perfectly good water for use in your lawn and garden. Rain barrels are great for urban environments and can be deployed by almost anyone with a small lawn, garden, or deck.

Bioswales are a slightly different animal. They are landscaping features designed with permeable gravel and compost to prevent buildup of sediment from rain events and to keep plants healthy. Bioswales capture rain, filter any contaminants, and direct the water back into the earth to replenish surface water bodies and groundwater systems.[12] Constructed bioswales can be gorgeous, and they require minimal maintenance.

Sustainable Home and Property Choices

For the Penny-Wiser	• When remodeling an existing home, pursue deconstruction rather than demolition. • Install a rain cistern to capture stormwater.
For the Be-Bester	• Dwell in a high-density structure for closer amenities and easy access to shops. • Preserve land through conservation measures.
For the Bridge Builder	• Purchase a pre-existing home. • Construct an accessory dwelling unit (ADU) on your home's property.
For the Nature Lover	• Turn a lawn or balcony into a certified wildlife sanctuary. • Install a xeriscape lawn plan.

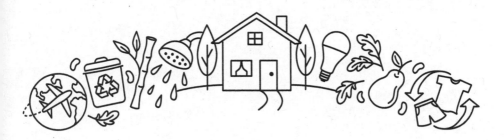

10

· · · · · · ·

Food

Tell me what you eat, and
I will tell you what you are.

JEAN ANTHELME BRILLAT-SAVARIN

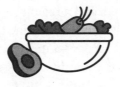

T WASN'T until I embraced the notion of becoming a "local" that my search for local foods became a passion. That began when I moved to Portland and decided to embrace a community-based life. I've had teachers along the way and wiser women who cajoled me along the path. Before Portland, you could say I lived an itinerant life, and proudly. Ever since I moved from my family home in northern Virginia to attend a rural college in New Hampshire, my life has been marked by change and movement. I lived in Boston for two years and then was off to Washington, DC, for three more. From there I moved to Philadelphia for twenty months, gaining my master's, and then onto NYC for twelve years. That last number is deceiving, though, because within that decade-plus, I moved four different times to three different neighborhoods and one new borough. Itinerant. That was the gig. During those intervening years, I dabbled with community-supported agricultural boxes and, most assuredly, was a frequent visitor to farmers markets, both DC's Eastern Market and NYC's Union Square Saturdays. And on several trips to the West Coast, I would make it a point to visit local farmers markets in the big cities of California. I basked in the diversity and bounty those markets provided as an East Coast interloper.

But, I was a shallow thinker when it came to food systems. A tinkerer in the moment, more delighted in the adventure and intrigue of a fun weekend hour outdoors than a woman on a mission to understand and raise up my local food community. That old Kate changed with my arrival in Oregon, a state with a rich, diverse natural ecosystem and a region blessed with outrageously fertile agricultural lands. Oregon is home to more than thirty-five thousand farms spread across 16 million acres of farmland, producing more than 220 commodity foods enjoyed by individuals across the globe.[1]

My passion project the first year living in Portland was to visit every local farmers market that ran in the warm months of spring and summer. That's not a simple feat in this "city of roses," where you can find at least one local street market in each of the inner-city Portland neighborhoods, bigger year-round markets like the Portland Farmers Market at Portland State University, and also sprawling local outdoor markets in the close-in suburbs of Portland proper. The city is a haven for craft purveyors of all types of food-stuff, from spelt breads, fresh canned jams, salsas, "fresh" (needing to be refrigerated) chocolates, and alternative milks, to even more niche products such as local, seasonally sourced dehydrated snacks and meals made by businesses like Fernweh Food Company. Like California, the Pacific Northwest is teeming with entrepreneurs who take the richness of the land seriously, as well as the health that well-grown, clean food can provide to individuals who seek to consume goodness directly from nearby soils.

Community-Supported Agriculture

Community-supported agriculture, simply known as CSA, is a membership-based model to financially support local farmers, cattle ranchers, and fishermen. CSA members—individuals and households—share in a farm's bounty by being supplied with locally produced, seasonally harvested food directly from it. Members commit to buying a box of produce consistently throughout the year, and, dependent on the type of CSA you become a member of, receive a pre-determined (or, in some cases, customized) mix of fruits, vegetables, meat, and fish. CSAs are an old concept that's been revived and reinvented for the modern age.

CSAs redevelop the relationship between producer and consumer, one that has been lost with the rise of industrialized agriculture, where food is grown in far-flung areas and seasonality is lost. The benefits are mutually reinforcing: farmers are supported by and develop a closer bond with the individuals they are feeding. There is an exchange of ideas, "wins," and rewards—and of unexpected crop bounties as well as intermittent failures. Farming struggles and successes are mutually shared. In turn, members gain the ability to eat ultra-fresh food and get to try unexpected seasonal crops with significantly lower carbon footprints, sourced within one hundred miles of where they live.[2]

My CSA is Hood River Organic, a farm located in the valley of Mount Hood, eighty-two miles directly east of Portland. I sign up for a box to be delivered every two weeks. I almost always go with the default fruit and vegetable picks because I know those are currently in season and, frankly, I dare myself to be surprised by items I've seen at the grocery store but have avoided for lack of knowing how to prepare them. My box arrives with loads of gorgeous beets with their leaves still intact; radiant chard and kale stalks; massive, gnarly celeriac roots; juicy, delicious apples and pears; and a constantly changing array of mushrooms, leafy greens, and fresh farm eggs. Unpacking the box is exciting, each and every time. I do have a brief moment of panic when my veggie drawers and refrigerator shelves are jam-packed with fresh produce and I'm unsure whether I can cook my way through this week's Earth's bounty, but I'm almost always rewarded with new inventions from researched recipes previously unknown and untried.

Meet Your Meat

Here's the skinny on animal meat: we eat too much as a nation. We do. I've been guilty of it for most of my life. I grew up in a family in which eating a balanced dinner necessarily meant having an equally portioned triumvirate of animal protein, a starch, and a

vegetable, preferably of the green variety. Every night. No excep-
tions! I carried that idea of "balanced" well into my thirties.

But eating meat has never been relegated to just the dinner
menu. We've been fed a steady diet of bacon on the weekends, as
well as sprinkled on our Cobb salads. We have sliced meat sand-
wiches for lunch, piled high. Here in Portland, our collective love
of meat expands to an obsession. It's the first city I've ever lived in
where you can find a parallel meat menu of specialty beef selec-
tions at a sushi restaurant. Meat in the US has become a garnish,
like parsley is in France and Pecorino cheese in Italy. Almost
every menu provides meat as an "additional" option to whatever we may desire to eat at that moment. Meat consumption has
almost become a nervous tick in our society. Meat?! Yes. Why?
Why not!

It's too much meat, though. We don't crave that much. Our bodies don't need that much. We overfeed ourselves animal protein
because, well, most of us were brought up on the idea that it was
the way to eat, especially if you could afford it.

Men and women need to consume, on average, 56 grams and
46 grams, respectively, of protein a day.[3] That doesn't mean it has
to be animal protein, just protein, and protein comes in a diverse
selection of options, including non-animal sources. Take a look at
these food groups, which individually and definitely in combination back a protein punch:[4]

- Legumes (or beans)
- Nuts
- Seeds (e.g., sesame, sunflower, and poppy)
- Specialty seeds (e.g., quinoa, chia, and amaranth)
- Hemp
- Soy products (e.g., tofu, tempeh, and edamame)
- Seitan (seasoned wheat gluten)

Why is there such a fuss about urging Americans to eat less
meat? There are three arguments in play. The first is an equity
argument: as the global population swells from some 7.5 billion
individuals today toward 11 billion people by the end of the century,

the amount of meat able to be produced for existing populations is already hitting against its upward limit. With the addition of more than 3 billion people on the planet, we must rationalize the protein needs of all and limit high-volume intake.

The second argument is one of environmental impact. Cattle production is feed-, land-, and water-intensive. Raising cattle for human consumption requires significant land for herds to roam. Cattle need to be fed and hydrated. The idea of using productive and increasingly limited agricultural lands to grow crops solely to make feedstock for animals doesn't make fundamental sense. And diverting fresh water for cattle versus human consumption is becoming an increasingly losing argument in a world where water availability and quality is diminishing exponentially from overuse and climate change impacts. Consider the following numbers:

- One-third of all arable land (or land suitable for producing food) is used for crop cultivation to feed livestock, not humans.[5]

- One-quarter of the planet's land surface is currently used for livestock grazing.[6]

- Almost three-quarters of the planet's freshwater resources are necessary for productive farming.[7] A large percentage of this water usage is attributed to livestock production.

- Nearly twenty percent of greenhouse gases in the atmosphere come from raising livestock for human consumption.[8]

Yikes! Is eating animals really that good for us?

The third argument is about our physical health. Eating industrialized meat, which entails feeding cattle a heavy diet of steroids and antibiotics, is detrimental to our bodies. It's a food chain issue. You and I are at the top of it. But whatever is placed into the bodies of the animals below us inevitably finds its way into our bodies, for better or worse. Would you shoot yourself up with steroids and antibiotics daily? Haven't we been told that steroids are bad for us? Yes, we have and yes, they are, in steady, persistent doses. Then why would you want to fill yourself up on a slab of sirloin steak that comes with a side of embedded steroids, just to "ooh and aah" about the flavor and taste?

The good news comes in many shapes and sizes. Meat and meat-like protein is plentiful here in the US. Our choices of what we eat, how much, and what type become a critical decision point for ourselves and the planet. I offer various perspectives below on how to source protein for your dietary consumption.

Meat CSAs

Just like fruit, vegetable, and grain CSAs, there are animal protein CSAs. My friend Diane Bradley, a Portland resident and transplant of Atlanta, Georgia, shares a meat CSA with another family. They purchase approximately twenty pounds of animal meat of different cuts and types, every month, netting each family ten pounds. Diane and her family enjoy the diversity of cuts and appreciate the relationship they have with the local farmers at Double F Ranch in Central Oregon. She can trust that the cattle and livestock have been treated humanely.

Community-Supported Fisheries

Individuals can also become members of CSFs, community-supported fisheries, where membership supports the livelihoods and living wages of local fishermen who harvest fair-trade, sustainable seafood from oceans and rivers close to your community.

Purchasing "Clean Meat" at the Grocery Store

The problem with labels is that they proliferate to the point of confusion. They start with a lack of standardization and grow muddier from there. But the alternative can be a murky business as well.

Meat without any classification of how it was raised and where it was sourced, and no details given about the farm or ranch from which the livestock came, can be even more telling. Beware of no labels. Understand the labels that designate meat as "clean": well cared for, not confined to stalls and defecating on themselves, having side-stepped being shot up with antibiotics and steroids to remain healthy before being slaughtered, and given food for fattening that we would be comfortable identifying as something recognizable in the natural environment.

Clean means that the meat you see and can purchase at the meat counter in any one of the many supermarkets you frequent in your town was fed real food, was treated humanely, and wasn't shot up with a cocktail of chemicals. Think about the choice between buying a bottle of Honest Tea with a hint of lemon and a can of Red Bull: they both will give you a jolt of energy, but one is made with ingredients you understand and know, and the other is a mixture of chemicals that can blister your mouth and erode the enamel of your teeth. Clean meat designates that for the life of the animal, the process of feeding and caring for it is one we can understand and recognize.

Think about purchasing meat that has the following labels:

- Hyper-local
- Hormone-free
- Antibiotic-free
- Organic
- Pasture-raised
- Humanely raised
- Grass-fed
- Non-GMO feed

Better yet, if your grocer can tell you the farm and the farmer that raised the meat and how far away they are located from where you are purchasing it, you can feel confident that those individuals stand by their farming practices. More importantly, it allows you to research who they are, what they stand for, and how they raise their livestock. Transparency does an educated consumer make.

Take pride in sourcing high-quality proteins. Although they may cost more than the average chicken leg, pork chop, or pound of cubed beef, you gain confidence in knowing that what you are deciding to ingest was raised well, contributing to your continued health.

Indeed, protein from meat sources and fish can help us meet our daily protein requirements easily. But a combination of three to five other protein alternatives can just as effectively get us to the right levels of daily protein intake without the need for meat and fish. If you are not gluten-free, seitan is a key go-to protein source in low quantities. If gluten must be avoided, a carefully selected combination of protein from nuts, seed, legumes, soy, and hemp can effectively (and with a diversity of options) get both men and women to their daily protein requirements. The reduction of GHG emissions from a strictly vegetarian or vegan diet equals sixty-three percent and seventy percent, respectively.[9] That may be sufficient incentive to embrace food consumption sustainability in your life from today forward!

Let me be clear: I am not advocating for you to adopt any extreme dietary measures. I'm an "everything in moderation" gal. Meat and fish are fantastic forms of protein for staying healthy and strong. The problem lies in our demand for animal protein. Demand has doubled over the last half-century with rising human populations and growing consumption levels that make "traditional" sources of protein from livestock and fish unsustainable. By mid-century, scientists estimate that meat production to meet human consumption demand would have to increase some seventy-six percent over today's levels, from 259 to 455 million tons annually.[10] A path forward to meet growing global demand via traditional cattle raising and feeding is not viable and certainly not environmentally sustainable.

TOM DOUGLAS

Protein hunter

NOT ALL of us, including myself, own a gun for hunting. I don't even know how to shoot. However, my fellow Dartmouth alum, Tom Douglas, does. Tom happens to be a senior scientist and cryospheric geochemist for the Department of Defense, studying Earth's processes in cold regions in order to apply those learnings in other harsh environments being affected by climate change impacts. He grew up in New Hampshire but has lived in Fairbanks, Alaska, for the last twenty-five years. We talked about all the ways in which he tries to mitigate his personal impact on the environment. When it comes to his food needs, he employs a region-centric and uniquely old-fashioned way to secure meat protein: he hunts moose once a year and fishes for salmon and halibut in local waters. He calls both proteins "clean" meat: sustainable, local, and organic sources that feed his family and his neighbors throughout the year. Tom estimates that he harvests about one hundred pounds of fish and two hundred pounds of moose meat each year, providing about a pound of meat daily for him and his daughter, with plenty to spare for others to enjoy. Except for buying eggs at his local grocer, he purchases very little additional animal protein.

Alternative Proteins

Guess what? It's a good time to be alternative... or just eat alternative proteins and "meats." Options abound and are increasingly more delicious by the day. Thankfully, their environmental impact on the planet is heavenly low compared to that of livestock.

Alternative proteins are vegetable-based meat substitutes enhanced in flavor and texture through the use of technology. These plant-based meats are presented in a way that imitates how animal protein is packaged today. It's a sleight of hand for individuals wary of alternative meats: "trick" individuals into trying protein alternatives by shaping them into meat forms that are familiar to us—hamburger patties, sausage links, and meat nuggets. The reality is a lot of people like the taste of animal meat: the juicy, fatty flavor that suffuses our mouths and fills our bellies.

The alternative protein space is exploding right now, for good reason. The cost of animal meat is rising, but so are the health scares from how that meat is harvested and made into food products to eat. Alternative protein brands are proliferating. I offer thoughts on three biggies below.

The brand Tofurky is generally considered the "father" of alternative protein, officially founded in 1980 by Seth Tibbott. Tofurky is the seitan king of alternative "meat." The company's packaging is fun and playful, and its meatless protein-packed products are found side by side with animal bacon, sausages, hot dogs, and hamburger patties in the refrigerator section of most grocery stores. Tofurky protein, when paired with meat fixings—ketchup, mustard, relish, onions, and peppers—has a comparable taste and texture to that of animal meat. Go ahead, try it!

Another, much younger start-up has made a splash in the alternative-meat space. Its name is Beyond Meat. The company's products are made from pea protein, engineered in the lab to mimic the taste profile, texture, and even "bleeding" capabilities of a perfectly crafted and cooked steak, hamburger, sausage, or pork cutlet. Beyond Meat is fast becoming a staple menu item at casual dining and fast-food restaurants across North America. You can walk into most McDonald's, KFC, Dunkin' Donuts, Carl's Jr., or Subway restaurants and order yourself a Beyond Meat hamburger, meatball sub, and breakfast sausage sandwich. But you don't need to eat fast food to enjoy Beyond Meat. Walk into your local grocery store and grab a twin-pack of hamburger patties ready to be grilled. I prefer Beyond hamburgers to the real beef kind. They are great tasting, especially ensconced in a P.F. Chang's–style lettuce wrap with tomato, pickles, and chipotle sauce on top. They're light in the mouth and give me no intestinal aftereffects that typically accompany a rich meat meal.

Impossible Foods is a direct rival of Beyond Meat and, by the nature of the alternative protein space, a near rival of Tofurky. Impossible's plant-based meats are made from fermenting soybean DNA in a genetically engineered yeast concoction. Basically, Impossible Burgers are made from genetically modified soybeans. Genetically modified means that the ingredients in Impossible's products have been engineered or altered from their original or natural state. Products made from GMO ingredients are controversial. I try to avoid them as much as possible. GMO products are banned in Europe because of concern with unintended consequences to the environment, natural biodiversity, and human health. Here in the US, GMO products are allowable and not well identifiable. Take a look at your Honey Nut Cheerios box. You'll find a small statement at the bottom of the narrow side of box that states, "Contains bio-engineered food ingredients," or GMO for those in the know.

Alternative proteins have some real benefits that ought to be championed:

- They require no cattle to be raised, fed, or slaughtered, thus avoiding the environmental pollution impacts from those activities.

- They can be engineered to include more protein, iron, and omega-3s while also avoiding the saturated fats found in naturally raised meat products.[11]

But you need to be diligent in understanding how the alternative meat substitutes you want and like to eat are being made. Remember what you value. If eating GMO products is a no-no for you, buy alternative proteins that are made from natural ingredients that have not had their DNA altered. Diligence, attention, and intention must forge a fierce bond.

Here's a final thought on alternative meats. A typical American adult eats 222 pounds of meat annually, or more than half a pound daily. That's nearly two and a half times what any other person on the planet consumes in a year. The average impact of an alternative meat product is 2.4 kilograms of carbon emissions per kilogram of product. Compare that to the environmental impact of traditional meat products (per equivalent kilogram):[12]

- Beef: 9 kg to 129 kg of carbon emissions
- Pork: 4 kg to 11 kg of carbon emissions
- Chicken: 2 kg to 6 kg of carbon emissions

Effectively, eating an alternative meat product is the equivalent to eating a small breast of chicken, the animal meat with the lowest carbon impact on the planet. So go ahead, eat your meat. Just make a conscious decision to start substituting alternative meats for those real ones.

New Meats: They're Going to Be "Real" Good

OK, I'm going to go scientific on you. Let's take a jaunt to the lab.

New meats go by many different names, not all psychologically palatable, but definitely edible. Here's a running list:

- Lab meat
- Clean meat
- Cultured meat
- Test-tube meat
- In vitro meat
- Cellular agriculture

New meat is protein grown in a laboratory from billions of cells cultured from skeletal muscle taken from the neck of a (real) cow. Those cells grow into muscle tissue that form the basis of meat harvested in a lab rather than from livestock on a farm. The process is complicated and requires scientists to grow not just meat cells but also fat cells (the fundamental basis for meat's taste), as well as to develop a circulatory system to deliver oxygen and nutrients to the meat and fat cells and to ensure metabolic waste is removed in the process.[13] This is why the commercial viability of lab meat is ten to twenty years away and likely to hit its stride as we near 2050. The thrill in the potential of lab meat is its near-zero environmental impact. Researchers who have made comparisons between the production of lab meat and traditional meat found huge climate change benefits to be gained:[14]

- 78–96 percent reduction in GHG emissions
- 7–45 percent reduction in energy use
- 99 percent lower land use
- 82–96 percent reduction in water consumption

These figures don't even address environmental pollution from chemical use that would be all but eliminated with the production of meat in laboratories to feed the world. Pesticides, fungicides, heavy metals, aflatoxins, melamine, anabolic agents, and antibiotics—all used in the raising of industrialized livestock and cattle feed—could be avoided.[15] Lab-grown meat is a technology that promises meat products derived from the cells of real meat that are clean (a.k.a. good) for the environment, healthy for humans, and abundant enough to feed the world. Is that enough of an argument to excite you?

Fishing for Change

Most of us know about farmed fish, right? We can either buy "fresh caught" fish or fish that's been farmed, which is fish protein cultivated for human consumption. The United Nations reports that approximately seventeen percent of the world's population (1.3 billion) depends on protein from fish (whether that be saltwater, freshwater, or shellfish) to meet their daily protein intake, so that's a lot of consumption.[16] Unfortunately, not all marine farming is good for the environment. In fact, many of the shrimp aquaculture farms found near coastal regions and close to estuaries are detrimental, destroying fragile ecosystems with waste and chemical pollution. These aquaculture systems also tend to overuse antibiotics to stave off disease while the fish are fattened.

Over the last ten years, there's been a movement toward developing deep ocean aquaculture farms, a sustainable form of fish farming using technologies to raise fish in the deepest reaches of the planet's oceans. Deep ocean aquaculture pods can be either floating or submerged marine cages, and they are becoming increasingly commercially viable. Norway's government just approved a floating marine pod off the coast of Trondheim for salmon farming, and both Panama and Mexico currently operate ocean farms for growing cobia and striped bass.[17] Deep ocean aquaculture seeks to avoid all the "bads" of land aquaculture farms while increasing the volume of fish farm production globally to meet the protein needs of the world's population:[18]

- Coastal ecosystems can go untouched or actively be restored.

- Pollution is much less of a concern given the size of the open ocean and the depths of the farms, which allow for dispersal and absorption of fish feed and waste.

- Antibiotics are minimally used because of the benefits of breeding fish in natural environments familiar to the populations being farmed.

The potential threat to biodiversity is still an open concern that needs to be addressed. Farm-bred fish can still escape ocean pods, although escapes are low for US aquaculture farms. The hope with deep ocean fishing is that many of the drawbacks of inshore aquaculture can be avoided altogether while "naturally" repopulating the oceans that have been drastically overfished during the last fifty years.

Fish, especially of the sustainably managed variety, is an excellent source of protein: rich in fatty acids, essential vitamins, and minerals; lean; and heart-healthy. A University of Oxford study from 2014 found that a pescatarian diet cut individual carbon footprints in half compared to those of individuals who relied on an animal-meat diet.[19] With sustainably managed deep-water aquaculture, there is hope of supplying the world with healthy, low-carbon, protein-rich fish in a way that side-steps the typical problems of farm fishing.

Sustainable Food Choices

For the Penny-Wiser	• Grow your own garden. • Consume one-quarter pound (one hamburger's worth) of meat or less per week, which will save you money and have less of an environmental and health impact.
For the Be-Bester	• Eat only seasonally grown food. • Become a vegetarian.
For the Bridge Builder	• Buy locally cultivated food. • Become a CSA member.
For the Nature Lover	• Follow a sustainable pescatarian diet. • Purchase non-GMO food products.

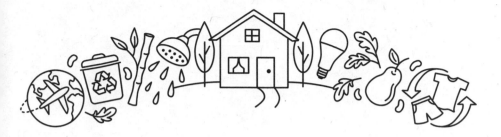

11

......

Material Goods

The good purchaser
devoted to "more,
newer, and better" was
the good citizen.

LIZABETH COHEN,
A Consumers' Republic

THE STUFF we buy helps to shape our personal identities: the tools and gadgets we use, the things we surround ourselves with, and what we put on our bodies. Much of that is simply consumed, such as beauty products, and what's left is the packaging, which ends up materially as trash, covered in Chapter 13. All manner of material goods—from consumables to soft goods, and electronics to large equipment—can be shared, which is discussed in Chapter 14. My background is in clothing manufacturing, and I've found that not only is clothing something we buy in great quantity, but it also serves as a proxy for all material goods. The broader themes found in a discussion on clothing—what materials make up the products we purchase, how the things we use are made, what happens to them after we're done with them, and what other options are available to us when we want or need more—can be applied to almost any good we use.

The Magic Trick That Turned Want into Need

There are very few "things" we need as humans to live a good and contented life. Abraham Maslow's hierarchy of needs tells that truth. In Maslow's hierarchy, the most essential elements required to support human happiness and contentment are "basic needs" that include access to sufficient food, water, warmth, and rest. Other basic needs include safety and security represented by the shelter of a home. Once these are met, the next set of needs we desire are psychological in nature; specifically, love and belonging. Nowhere in Maslow's hierarchy does he identify material wealth or the consumption of an abundance of products as a basic human "need." I'd argue that a fifth pair of sneakers, a drawer full of personal electronic gadgets, or a fleet of vehicles does not make us more secure.

Peer pressure, societal perceptions, and psychological triggers that are deftly pulled by advertising firms through compelling phraseology and visually audacious digital storytelling play on our sense of wants desired by transforming them into needs required. We easily fall prey to these forces and justify our consumption of products by mirroring the messages we've absorbed through mass media exposure.

Why NOT *buy those shoes? They're twenty-five percent off.*

I signed up for a monthly makeup box subscription because I deserve a little pampering.

My son's obsessed with LEGO *and he gets bored easily. I buy him a couple of building sets every week to keep him occupied.*

Shopping is so easy online. With Amazon Prime, I can order almost anything and have it arrive by noon the next day.

We as consumers are lulled either subliminally or overtly, and reassured that yes, in fact we do absolutely need what we desire right now—ideally, yesterday—because it will make us prettier, handsomer, sexier, cooler, funnier, more popular, and special.

Remember Tiffany & Co.'s successful advertising campaign targeted to single women?

> Your left hand sees red and thinks roses. Your right hand sees red and thinks wine. Your left hand believes in shining armor. Your right hand thinks knights are for fairy tales. Your left hand says, "I love you." Your right hand says, "I love me, too." Women of the world, raise your right hand.

The ad suggests being an independent woman very much means you should indulge yourself with expensive jewelry purchases.

The more insidious forms of "advertising" can be found in personal electronics. Think about the annual rollouts hyped by the media and overwritten about by journalists covering industry trends and technology "advancements": the "new, upgraded, most innovative, never-before-unveiled"—wait for it—smartphone, tablet, computer, laptop, or video game. Apple has been one of the biggest perpetrators of this methodology and the most successful at it. No sooner would the company announce the new iteration of the iPhone and its formal release date at one of the many technology conferences, and people would be lining up outside stores, waiting for the doors to fling open so they could be the first to purchase the new gadget.

Never mind the new technology may not be significantly different than the previous year's. Never mind the items could cost thousands of dollars more the first day than just three months later. Never mind those who waited in line likely didn't need the newest version. They *wanted* it, and that was enough. For these early adopters, they need the new technology because having it reinforces internalized notions of who they consider themselves to be: innovators, sophisticated technologists, the coolest gadget geeks. They could claim some level of superiority over others just based on being in possession of the newest iPhone.

We've been told to consume in America, because consuming has been interwoven into how we are supposed to see, be, and feel about ourselves. And detrimentally, we are told incessantly to loathe what is natural. Your hair color? Not brown enough. Your eyelashes? Not long or thick enough. Those laugh lines on your face? Ugly. Your underwear? Not the right kind to lift, fill, tuck, and tighten.

The messages bombarding us to consume are insidious. They hijack our deepest fears and concerns. We are told to consume so as to avoid the nightmarish fates we fear deep down in our subconscious. We consume because we are told, in so many words and images, that buying this and that will make our life better, fuller, richer. Remember the commercial for Dos Equis beer, "The Most Interesting Man in the World"? Drink Dos Equis and you too can become the most interesting man in the world. Or so the not-so-subliminal message goes.

We don't necessarily intellectually believe in the stated (or unstated) causality between purchasing something and gaining an attribute or acquiring an identity, but the idea of its potentiality is seductive. "Why not?" we say to ourselves. Maybe buying these things will make me fun, flirty, and irreverent ... or some better version toward my ideal self.

Having more things does not make us better humans. Buying more consciously and more sustainably makes us better citizens. Consuming products that have a low or no impact on the environment should be the more desirable way to buy. You know what's really cool? Consuming responsibly.

I ask you: try to understand how peer pressure affects your buying desires, how psychological triggers in advertising sway you. Acknowledge that the system of consumption here in the US is very much a post–World War II construct. Awareness builds our capacity for change. And changing the way we consume is critical, not just from a moral but also a sustainability standpoint. We must seek to reduce and reverse our personal impact on the planet.

You Are What You Wear

Do you know what the shirt you are wearing is made of? How about your pants, sweater, or jacket? When it gets cold outside and you decide to don a hat and some gloves, what materials make up those items? Look at the clothing labels. Can you decipher what the materials are and whether they come from natural sources or are synthetically made?

The textile industry has so many new names for different types of fibers and fabrics that this particular lack of knowledge is understandable. And yet, what our sheets, furniture, carpets, and clothes are made from is fundamentally important to you and the planet.

Most of what we buy today—I'm talking seventy percent or more of our clothes, sheets, and furniture—is made using polyester fibers. Refined fossil fuels. Can you imagine? Think about that for a minute. It's not pleasurable to have these products on your body for long periods of time. Skin doesn't like fossil fuels near it. It gets itchy and irritated. Polyesters are allergenic, an irritant. Every time you wash a piece of polyester clothing, it pills and sloughs off microplastics that wash into the sewage system and out to our oceans and rivers to contaminate our natural environment. Every wash. The microplastic pollution contribution alone from polyester materials is enormous.

Natural, renewable fibers and fabrics are good for our bodies and have a soft impact on the planet. Natural fibers derive from materials produced by or found in nature—such as trees, cotton, or grass—that grow quickly without the need for fertilizers and pesticides.[1] They tend to have embedded beneficial properties that are bestowed to the product users. They can be antimicrobial, antiallergen, highly moisture-absorbent, breathable, durable, and antistatic, to name a few.

A Quick Chat about Jeans

Jeans are a purely American invention, albeit by an immigrant from Germany. They were made to be worn by working men. Levi Strauss went into business with the customer who ordered a pair of these sturdy, durable pants for himself, Jacob W. Davis.[2] Those jeans and the ones that followed for the next one hundred years were made from one hundred percent cotton, embellished with a few copper rivets and some brass buttons. Today, the jean has been "innovated." It is difficult to find a pair of jeans made solely from cotton fiber. Jeans and most clothing items sold today are cotton blends: the natural cotton fiber has been interwoven with a synthetic or man-made fiber. We know cotton comes from cotton plants even though we may not exactly understand the process of converting a cotton boll into a fiber and yarn for making clothes and home furnishings. Whereas knowing where synthetic materials come from is far less understood. It's complicated, too.

Take your favorite pair of jeans. Mine is the LA brand AG, short for Adriano Goldschmied. Do you love your jeans? I do. I love the washes with the fake creases at the front hip corners. I like the height of the jeans, which accommodate my chubby short waist. I like how the jeans feel. The AG jeans I buy are a cotton blend, made with two percent Lycra material, which provides just enough give. How about yours?

Here's the problem. Jeans of old, like the Levi Strauss ones I exclusively wore into my mid-thirties, were made from one hundred percent cotton. They didn't have any designed give to them. The give came from wearing the jeans repeatedly for months. The whole idea of jeans back then was that you "broke" them in and contoured them to your body through years of wear. And they literally lasted for years. I remember holding on to my pairs of jeans for a decade or more. I would have had them longer if I hadn't, ahem, gained weight and grown out of them.

Now, with cotton blends euphemistically called "stretch denim," jeans don't last. I know. My AG jeans stop looking hot on my bod after about two years of wear. They start to sag in all the wrong places, like the crotch, butt, and knees. Annoying. I first thought this happened because I was washing them too often. Or had I lost weight? (Oh, how I wish!) Then, I understood after reading an explanation about denim repair on a jeanmaker's website:

> While we can repair nearly any type of jeans, we mostly work on virgin (raw) denim. Why? Because at a certain point in time, generally after multiple years of wear, stretch denim will reach the end of its lifespan, as it will have become too thin or stretched out to repair.[3]

Jeans made from one hundred percent cotton can last a decade or more. Stretch denim jeans? Two or three years at the most, unless you like sags in all the important places.

Synthetic Textiles

Man-made or synthetic fibers are created in a lab. There is a class of synthetic fibers that transform natural plant and wood pulp into fabrics that remain commercially biodegradable. You may be familiar with some of those branded names: Lyocell, rayon, Modal, acetate.

Clothing made from Modal, a cellulose fiber made from wood pulp, is particularly coveted for its softness and how it bounces back to its original shape post-wash. Even though these fibers are man-made, their base materials come from naturally occurring sources and retain many of their beneficent attributes.

There is another growing class of synthetic fabrics derived not from natural materials but from fossil fuels finding their way into clothing and home goods. We grew up with nylon; that synthetic fiber is as common to us as apple pie. But there are many other synthetics going under generic or branded monikers: acrylic, polyester, spandex, Lycra, Gore-Tex, Kevlar, and DrySport, to name a few. There is a boom in the manufacture of synthetic fabrics. Seventy percent of all fibers made in the world today are man-made fibers, sixty percent of which are polyester-based. And that's bad. Polyester-based fabrics are made from—can you guess it? Fossil fuels, namely natural gas and oil.

So the volume of clothing being produced for global consumption is growing exponentially because of the emergence of just-in-time manufacturing and the adoption of "fast fashion." That growth in consumer products is almost entirely fueled by new synthetic fabrics.[4]

Cotton fabric makes up thirty percent of all fiber made and used today. Global demand for synthetic fabrics is projected to grow nearly four percent year over year for the foreseeable future.[5] And, yep, you guessed it: the demand for polyester is massive. Too bad for us that polyester blends are non-biodegradable, non-recyclable forms of fabric that contribute big-time to climate change.

Let's get back to those blends in clothing that are becoming more typical, increasingly manufactured by brands and purchased and worn by individuals. Once a clothing blend goes over a small threshold, such as a blend containing more than five percent synthetic material, that particular piece of clothing's recyclability drops to zero.

Let's look at that another way. A one hundred percent cotton T-shirt can technically be thrown into a commercial composting bin and biodegrade back to regenerate Earth's soils. Put aside the fact that most of us do not compost our clothing. Now, technically, a button-down blouse made from one hundred percent linen could also be composted if, say, we stripped it of its plastic buttons. Jeans made of one hundred percent cotton could also enjoy the same fate if we stripped away the brass rivets and metal zipper from the cotton. But once a company moves away from manufacturing clothing with natural fibers (e.g., cotton, wool, silk, hemp, linen) and introduces a synthetic and likely polyester fiber derived from natural gas and oil, the recyclability of that garment becomes wishful thinking.

The growth in and our dependence on synthetic polyester fibers just amplifies our consumption problem. We went from buying too much of naturally made products to consuming too much of really bad-for-the-earth things. We now have created a compounding problem because of our growing appetite for things that require natural resources (cotton, wool, water, and land) that are in limited supply, are fossil fuel derived, degrade our environment, and are not recyclable. Whether the fibers come from natural or synthetic sources, the textile industry is not kind to our water resources. It takes over five hundred gallons of water to make one pair of jeans, for instance.[6] And the amount of hazardous chemicals used in the production of fabric and finished goods is immense and highly dangerous to human and marine species. Water used during the dyeing and finishing processes is infused with hundreds of toxic chemicals that are then flushed out of factories and into bodies of water that they end up contaminating. But synthetics derived from oil and gas create even more problems.

Carbon Emissions of Synthetics

The entire global textile industry is a huge carbon emitter; it generates eight percent of the world's carbon emissions annually, in fact.[7] Polyester-type synthetic clothes are a key driver of the industry's carbon emissions number.

The very fact that synthetic fibers are derived from petroleum, a fossil fuel, tells us that a significant amount of energy was expended extracting oil from the ground, as well as in the technical transformation of producing polymers to form yarn to spin into clothing. The Stockholm Environment Institute studied how much carbon was emitted into the atmosphere per one metric ton of fiber spun for the most common fabrics used in textiles today. The findings for two—cotton and polyester—are shown in the following graph:

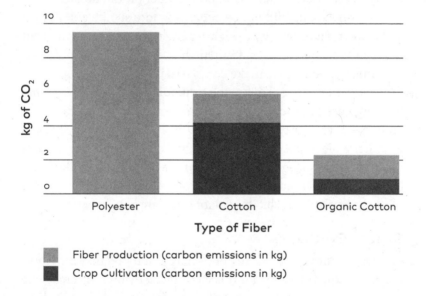

Total Carbon Emissions (kg/MT of Fiber)

SOURCE: Nia Cherrett et al., *Ecological Footprint and Water Analysis of Cotton, Hemp and Polyester* (Stockholm Environment Institute: Stockholm, 2005), 14.

In the polyester bar, you'll notice there's no amount for crop cultivation. There are no carbon emissions for "cultivating" polyester because it is made from gas and oil, not harvested plants. Also note how much higher polyester's carbon emissions from fiber production are. This is because the "materials" that go into making polyester have to be mined and blasted, refined, and chemically transformed into a fiber in order to have yarn spun to make a finished clothing piece. All of those activities are energy- and emissions-intensive in comparison to cotton plants that need water and sunlight to grow. Both cottons are some forty to seventy-five percent less carbon-intensive than the man-made polyester.

Energy Intensity of Synthetics

Turning cotton into yarn takes less than half (forty-five percent) the energy required to convert petroleum into polyester.[8] If we were to compare the energy intensity of cotton fiber production to that of acrylic or nylon, the difference becomes more significant. Acrylic and nylon require seventy to eighty percent more energy than cotton. Synthetic fibers, no matter which ones you are talking about, demand more energy to make compared to natural fibers.

This exercise in looking at the embodied energy—the amount of energy used at each step of the production and manufacturing process—of various types of fabrics is meant to show that what you wear has a big impact on your individual carbon emissions. Clothing and home soft-good products made from natural fibers are better for the environment, produce less carbon emissions, last longer, are recyclable and biodegradable, and are better for our health.

Cost of Synthetics

Although naturally fabricated goods may cost more, they are worth the extra expense. Consider this example: a nylon rug versus one made from wool. A synthetic nylon rug is relatively inexpensive ($2 to $15/yard versus $5 to $26/yard for wool) and easy to make. But it doesn't last as long as a wool rug. Depending on the quality and use of a nylon rug, its lifespan is anywhere between four and nine years. A wool rug will last a lifetime. Cleaning wool requires maintenance and care, but its durability is superior to any synthetic alternative. An inexpensive price may be enticing at first blush, but it's worth noting that old adage that holds true even today: You get what you pay for.

A Final Word on Synthetics

We are not always going to be able to avoid buying synthetic fibers, especially if we are avid mountain climbers, skiers, sailors, and race-car drivers, to name a few sporting activities where technical fibers allow us to remain dry in very wet conditions, stay warm in extreme weather, and keep from bursting into flames during collisions where fuel is in close proximity. Technical fibers are technological advancements that often serve a beneficial purpose. But, for most normal, everyday circumstances, a synthetic product often has a better natural substitute.

What's Old Is New Again

Our system of consuming material things is changing, whether we realize it or not. Little sparkles of transformation are occurring across the spectrum of consumer brands. Think of them as apparel industry will-o'-the-wisps; enticing orbs of light that lead those who follow away from the beaten path.

To rethink how we consume and to have companies provide alternate modes of use, reuse, and renewal in the apparel industry is revolutionary. Below I share three distinct examples of new business models that help you consume less clothing and in a different way.

The Reality of Clothing Recycling

Historically, when it came to "recycling" clothing, there were three possible paths to pursue. The first option was to cut or rip up our old clothing, sheets, and towels, and reuse them as rags for mopping up kitchen spills, Windexing our windows, or washing the car. In corporate sustainability speak, this is a "downcycling" option: taking something of quality and transforming it into something of lesser quality but with some retained value.

The second option would be to hand down clothing to a younger sibling, neighbor, or friend. I can't tell you how many of my older brother's clothes I wore through my elementary and middle school years. Maybe it's because of all the boy clothes I wore that I identified as a tomboy. Hand-me-downs become such because we know innately that clothes have a certain useful life, and that use doesn't end with their first owner. This is a classic "reuse" model of consumption. Consume a product until its inherent or perceived value has been used up or exhausted.

The third recycling option that has become society's option of choice is to donate our clothing to Goodwill, the Salvation Army, or some other similar organization. Donating makes us feel good, right? We're told it's the right thing to do so that what we no longer want, need, or, more fundamentally, value avoids our trash bin and, hopefully, meets with a new life outside of our realm of influence. That's generally true, but not in the way you may think.

You and I over the course of a year will seek to get rid of around eighty pounds of clothing. If you have a nine-year-old living in your house, pick that little guy up right now. He weighs the equivalent of all those unwanted clothes. If you are not a clothing-donating kind of person, almost all of your old clothes (ninety-five percent) will be thrown in your trash bin to be deposited in a landfill, even though sixty-eight pounds of it could have been successfully recycled.[9] That's kind of a bleak number. But this one that comes next may dishearten you even more.

Up to ninety percent of all clothing deposited in donation bins and given to charities goes . . . where? To clothing recyclers.[10] Not to new owners to be worn again (and again and again). Clothing recyclers sort and separate clothing into "like" materials and blends, then cut, shred, and package the material to be sold to downcyclers—there's that word again—to be used to mop up industrial waste, become a filler material for carpet pads or insulation, be re-spun into yarn, or be made into paper.[11] Of the ninety percent of clothing that is donated by you and me, half of it is essentially downcycled into fillers and rags for industrial or commercial purposes.[12] The other half is baled by the clothing recyclers and shipped far afield, to poor African and Asian countries to be sold to their citizens for nickels and pennies. And yes, the individuals in those countries get to wear the clothing that you donated, but the downside of this is that those countries are inundated with merchandise they likely don't want, that was not locally made, and that fundamentally undercuts their home-grown economies. And let's be real, all that shipping of shirts, pants, sweaters, coats, and shoes you don't want any more halfway across the globe is not great from an emissions standpoint. Your old clothing that was well-intentionally donated had to be shipped to a recycler somewhere in the US, who then sorted and baled items to be flown or sailed to far-off places, where they were trucked to a local market before they reached their potential new owners. It's crazy-making, in an *Alice in Wonderland*, upside-down-is-right-side-up sense.

Let's just say this: our donation system is inundated with unwanted stuff, and essentially broken. However, here's where the tiny lights of transformation in the clothing industry start to get exciting.

Renewed Clothing

There are companies here in the US working with a small but growing list of clothing brands that are intervening in this trash-or-donate conundrum. Eileen Fisher is a good example of a brand that is building a market and drumming up demand for "renewed" clothes. Renewed clothing to Eileen Fisher is clothes that were initially bought new, worn and loved by someone, and then sent back to the brand to be refurbished—holes mended, style rejuvenated, cleaned, tagged for resale—and sold again to a new (sustainably minded) buyer. This clothing retains the brand name and carries the same cachet as newly manufactured clothes, but at a lower price point. Renewed clothing side-steps the stigma of donated clothing as being cast-offs or of low value. It also extends the brand to new buyers who value the aesthetic, quality, and sustainable story of the clothing articles but may not be able to afford the price point of newly made clothes. The companies helping brands like Eileen Fisher renew clothing for secondary resale include The Renewal Workshop and Trove. They work directly with clothing brands to refurbish and repackage clothing to look like new at an attractive price. Going back to my corporate speak for one more second, this type of recycling is called "upcycling": creating the same quality product as the original.

KATHERINE DEUMLING

A "new" renewed clothing customer

MY FRIEND Katherine Deumling, a German transplant to the Pacific Northwest, former Slow Food USA chairwoman, current entrepreneur of Cook with What You Have, and minor Portland celebrity, shops Eileen Fisher's Renew clothing. She had always admired the style and quality of clothing the brand made, but Eileen Fisher's price point was out of reach for Katherine. In 2009, the brand launched Green Eileen, which was a clothing take-back program that cleaned, repaired, and resold not-new clothing at a discount. The program transformed into its Renew program and allowed Katherine to become a rabid Eileen Fisher clothing loyalist. She swears by the brand and its clothing and counts herself lucky to be able to afford a luxury brand because of its Renew program.

The Service Model of Manufacturing

Do you remember, back in the day, when brands and most department stores offered free alterations on new clothing purchases? My days of walking into Brooks Brothers with my dad so he could purchase a new blazer or suit are seared into my memory. I remember sitting on the carpeted step inside the dressing room in front of a three-way mirror so the tailor could right-size his pant cuffs or make fine adjustments to the suit jacket in the shoulders, waist, and sleeves. Those were the days. Well, maybe not, because I found the women's section of Brooks Brothers stuffy and conservative. It may be why the brand filed for bankruptcy. Who wears formal work clothes when we've transitioned to wearing "soft" pants with a presentable top to conduct video calls?

Tailoring and alterations have not necessarily gone away entirely. Many department stores still offer the services, whether for full-priced clothing purchases or special "club" members for free or a fee. But it's relatively rare these days. Why? You can blame fast fashion and our throwaway culture. Who keeps a suit for more than a season or two these days? Back then, suits were a decade-long proposition.

But the idea of offering alterations on clothing items is an old one that I'm starting to see be reinvented in modern ways.

Denham is a men and women's clothing manufacturer and retailer headquartered in Amsterdam. The company was founded on the idea of making high-quality jeans and knitwear. What is so intriguing about the brand is that it decided early on, as part of its business model, to be both a manufacturer and service provider for its clothes. Denham sells its clothing at its own branded stores. Additionally, it operates "Denim Bars," where individuals—whether customers of Denham or not—can go to request a jean repair, a reinforcement sew, a new wash, an embellishment, or desired embroidery, all for a fee. That's the key: the fee. This service model of manufacturing is a new concept for consumer brands, but one that makes really smart economic and material value sense. By employing this manufacturing "model," companies can make fewer new products by servicing what currently exists in the marketplace.

From the perspective of consumers, there is pride in owning a product that continues to retain value. I love my jeans. If you love your jeans, you want to keep wearing them. Denham loves them too and lovingly works to ensure their longevity and value for you.

I keep getting back to that word: value. Something valuable is loved and appreciated.

Revalorizing Clothing

Which leads me into my final transformative idea: revalorizing clothing to be "new" again. The idea of making old clothing into brand-new, pristine, "virgin" items is not commercial; not today. But it will be. It has the potential to transform our system of material use, which has a serious attendant problem: trash.

A company in Seattle, Washington, is working on this very initiative. Its name is Evrnu. It's a technology company, specifically one that has developed a patented series of processes to dissolve clothing into a pulp or cellulose slurry and then reconstitute that base material to make brand-new, high-quality clothing. Cool, right?

Currently, the company has the ability to do this with all types of blended materials. Its immediate focus is on making its technology available to clothing recyclers of ninety-five percent or higher cotton blends. The trick—it's not a trick but hard, worthy work—is to turn the clothing industry on its head. To do that, the Evrnus of the world have to work with all of the companies that handle old clothing: the clothing we're done with after we've used it, abused it, loved it, and tossed it. If Evrnu can convince clothing recyclers to sort out clothing that is made from at least ninety-five percent cotton, install its NuCycl technologies for processing those clothing items, and then sell the reconstituted fiber to yarn and fabric makers to weave the NuCycl cotton material into fabrics used to make new clothing, we can effectively stop cotton clothing from entering the trash cycle.

That's a big "if." But the concept of fully recycling cotton back into the fibers of new clothing is not a matter of if but when. And that is just the start of this idea. We tackle and conquer cotton, and we move on to the nylons and polyesters of the world. This new system of operating is one where old clothes are regenerated into new ones through a process of isolating the base materials that are used to make our clothing—cotton, wool, natural gas, oil—and reconstituting them in such a way that the core value of the materials is retained. We continue to recognize the material value of items even after our personal interest in them has waned, and we sidestep the trash heap.

Sustainable Material Goods Choices

For the Penny-Wiser	• Use Swedish reusable cellulose-based "paper towels." • Switch to waxed cotton food wraps to preserve foods in the refrigerator.
For the Be-Bester	• Buy sustainably made soft goods. • Buy all-natural products.
For the Bridge Builder	• Bring your own glass containers to restaurants for doggy-bagging. • Buy used, refurbished, or revalorized durables (e.g., computers) and soft goods (e.g., couches).
For the Nature Lover	• Buy "renewed" clothing. • Buy paper sandwich and snack bags.

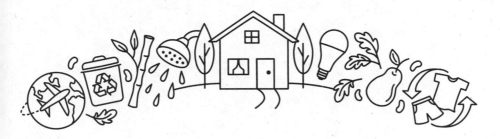

12

······

Water

No water, no life.
No blue, no green.

SYLVIA EARLE

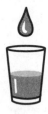

HOW WE think about and casually use water in our homes is another area where small, routine changes create impactful freshwater sustainability habits. Vast gallons of fresh water literally flush down our drains with minor to no contamination, never to be used again. Shower and bathroom faucet water funnels into the same municipal sewage system—or black pipes—to ultimately be cleaned, filtered, and discharged into river, lake, and ocean bodies. It is an unnecessary waste of fresh, drinkable water.

From outer space, Earth is this marbled blue-green beauty of a sphere, dotted with green and brown landmasses and sprinkled within massive stretches of blue oceans and seas. You know the numbers. Seventy-one percent of the planet is covered in water. The oceans contain some ninety-seven percent of all the water found on Earth. But salt water cannot be readily consumed by humans. We would need to desalinate salt water to make it available for us to drink. Humans can only consume fresh water. Drinkable—potable—water is found in lakes, rivers, creeks, and underwater aquifers. Fresh water is also found in glaciers and ice caps (think Mount Everest and the Rockies), but these last two sources are hardly accessible to us. I'm not sure I've ever heard someone remark to me, "I'm taking a trip to Mount Rainier to chip away at a glacier there so I can heat up a pot of water to make pasta tonight."

The water we drink mostly comes from lakes and reservoirs and from water from snow melt that runs downhill in the spring and summer months through mountains and forests and into rivers and streams. We also get our water from below the surface of the earth.

We "tap" that water by drilling wells and pulling it out through a pulley and lever system.

One percent. That's effectively the water that's readily available for humans to drink.[1] Doesn't seem like a lot, does it? Seven and a half billion people need access to fresh water to drink, cook, and wash. Do we have enough fresh water for everyone to drink, cook, and clean with?

- 1.1 billion people worldwide lack sufficient access to fresh water.

- 2.7 billion experience a month where fresh water is scarce or intermittently available.

- 2.4 billion people lack adequate water to stay clean.[2]

"Phew," you might say, "thank goodness fresh water is readily available here in America. It runs right out of my home faucets. No worries. And I don't pay a lot for my water. It's not an expense that makes me worry or keeps me up at night."

However, not only is fresh water precious, but it takes energy to pipe it into our homes so that it flows seamlessly through our faucets and showers and washes away the contents of our toilets, washing machines, and dishwashers. In fact, across the whole of the US, six percent of carbon emissions come from moving water to its final destination.[3] If you live in California, twenty percent of the state's total carbon emissions come from pumping water to homes, businesses, and farms.

Also, there is a complacency in seeing what infrastructure exists currently for us but not for others. There is a false sense of comfort in taking for granted water that so easily flows with a turn of a nozzle. We cannot take our freshwater resources for granted. Large swaths of the US are currently categorized as "water-stressed regions" because demands for water are high, groundwater aquifers are drying up and not being replenished fast enough to meet annual withdrawals, and climate change impacts, namely multi-year droughts, zap the land's ability to support the water demands of individuals, towns and cities, agricultural growers, and industry.

America is rich in natural resources. It is well endowed with goodness. But natural resources can diminish. Water can become scarce... and not just temporarily. Water quality can go from good to deadly. Talk to the residents of Flint, Michigan, site of a man-made disaster that challenged our belief that natural is better than treated. In 2014, the city of Flint made a cost-savings move to supply its residents with "natural" water from the Flint River instead of water treated by the municipality. After ongoing complaints of foul smells, discoloration, and a bad taste, it was discovered that the water from the Flint River was making people sick. The not-so-secret news was that the Flint River had been used as an open sewer, an industrial chemical dumping ground, for decades. Shocker: nature can't take care of itself if we override and overwhelm its natural systems!

Our freshwater resources are under threat from a dual menace: climate change and man-made impacts. Knowing that, we must consider how and how much we use water in our lives. Taking steps to decrease the quantity of water we use sets us up to build our sustainability muscle so that we begin to more fully value and quantify the resources we use.

Sitting Pretty

I've gotta ask you an uncomfortable question. How many times do you think you use the toilet each day? The entire day, from prone, eyes open, to head-on-the-bed asleep. Five times? Eight times?

I feel like I need to either release or evacuate my bodily fluids some dozen times a day. I was born with a small bladder, and then that vessel got wrecked from birthing two kids. I know, TMI.

An average person flushes the toilet after a jaunt to the bathroom ten times a day. If that flush is taking place on a non-efficient toilet, seven gallons of water are used for every flush.[4] So, on average, seventy gallons of water are needed per person per day. Over the course of a year, one person could have used some twenty-six thousand gallons of water to flush down each iteration of their number ones and twos. Multiply that by the number of people in your immediate family and we start getting into some very big numbers.

The water we use adds up, or in this case, flushes down to commingle with other "fluids" held in our sewer system. Every single gallon of water we are talking about is typically of the freshwater kind, meaning the precious one percent of all available water found on Earth that is readily drinkable by humans. You may ask yourself, "Why are we using fresh water—the drinkable kind—to flush away bodily fluids?"

This discussion prompts another question: Have you ever thought about not flushing your toilet after a tinkle? Instead of flushing every time you make a trip to the toilet, how about every other time? Especially if we are talking about the proverbial number-one release.

I get it. It might feel weird, keeping a pale yellow bowl of diluted urine around the house until the next bathroom visit. But it really is a thing people do. I do. And so do others around the globe. Diluted urine doesn't smell that much. We could see it as something waiting for additional concentration, so to speak.

Think about it: Why not *not* flush every time we go pee if we can halve our freshwater usage when using the toilet? It feels like a no-brainer to me.

Here's my story for how I got my head around the idea of not flushing as often as every toilet run. It goes back to my NYC days. I am a yoga practitioner. After visiting many studios in the city, the Jivamukti Yoga Center (now closed) became my go-to practice location. It was there where I first read this little ditty, which was posted on the inside of each bathroom stall for "sitters" to contemplate privately in a very public, high-traffic setting: "If it's yellow, let it mellow. If it's brown, flush it down." *Hmm*, I thought, *interesting*. The founders of Jivamukti, Sharon and David, were asking the collective of yoga adherents to consider not flushing pee when each of us goes wee.

Curiously, the phrase came up the other day when I was reading a 2019 *Time* magazine article on Cape Town's shrinking water supply due to three years of extreme drought conditions:

> The city has capped household water usage at eighty-seven liters (twenty-three gallons) per person, per day. For most homes, that means keeping showers under 2 minutes, no watering the garden or washing the car, refraining from flushing the toilet unless absolutely necessary, recycling bathing water where possible, and severely limiting dishwasher and washing machine use. Water storage tanks are already on backorder, unwashed hair is now a symbol of upright citizenship, and public restrooms are festooned with admonishments to "*let it mellow.*" [5]

Contrary to popular belief and standard practice in the US, not every trip to the bathroom needs a flush. There are many effective ways to mask odors, if you are worried they will arise. And if you find yourself game for a try, I leave you with a tip that works in my house. Transparency comes in handy with friends who visit or are deciding to encamp at your home. Tell them about your family practice and why it's important to you. You may get the same reaction as I did from my friends. When I informed a recent house guest of our practice, she replied nonchalantly, "Yep, I get it. I do it too in my house. I'm from California, remember?"

JILL SUGHRUE

Progress over perfection

JILL IS a sixty-six-year-old grandmother of two. She's been married to her husband, Patrick, for twenty-eight years. They own a super-insulated 2,500-square-foot house that they hand-built in 1998 on one acre. Jill jokes that she was a conservative Democrat and Patrick was a liberal Republican when they met nearly thirty years ago. Over the years they have aligned on sustainability and today both consider themselves solid Democrats.

Jill said that her "eyes were opened" after she and Patrick participated in a Voluntary Simplicity discussion course offered by Northwest Earth Institute in 1994. The course provided simple lessons on how to consciously buy products and personal challenges around supporting social equity and natural resource conservation. In addition to buying organic, driving an electric vehicle, and reducing waste, Jill consciously pursues water-saving measures. Jill learned via their water bill that she and Patrick use about five cubic feet of water per day (approximately thirty-eight gallons). Compare that to the average American, who uses between eighty and one hundred gallons of water per day. Jill and Patrick employ the following water-saving practices:

- They do not water the lawn.

- They do not flush every single time.

- They try to limit showers to five minutes.

- They put dishes in the sink and allow the water from hand washing to soak them.

- They only wash dishes and clothes when there's a full load.

- Leftover drinking water in glasses is used to water plants.

So Many Types of Water: Black, Gray, Blue, and Green

For most of my life, I thought about water in just two ways: fresh and salt water. Fresh water was water I could put in my mouth and swallow without a worry. Salt water was ocean water that technically could be swallowed, but wasn't drinkable.

Blue Water

I grew up vacationing in Sandbridge, an extended public-private coastal community of Virginia Beach. I loved playing and swimming in the ocean and surfing the waves. I drank a lot of ocean water in my day, but not willingly. It came about as a result of getting tumbled in the waves and mixed about in the underwater sands. Mostly, playing in the ocean was thrilling and, occasionally, scary. Those latter times when I walked out of the surf breathless, sandy-faced, with hair tousled and my bathing suit slightly askew, the full force of Earth's oceans, the power of its waves and the cycle of its tidal system, awed me.

We know and identify with "blue" water. That's water found in bodies both fresh and salt. Most blue water is available for our recreational pleasure but does not support our body's system. The bad news is that the process of water desalination is energy-intensive, and the technology to convert bad "blue" water into the good drinkable kind is expensive in large quantities. Hence, while desalination technology exists and is being deployed in water-scarce regions such as the Middle East and in highly populous, water-poor states such as Texas and California, it's not available at the scale needed to supply drinkable water as readily and voluminously as we have come to expect water to be here in the US.

Blue water is not the only type of water we should be aware of.

Gray Water

Gray water is slightly used water: those droplets that run down shower drains and out of bathroom faucets, dishwashers, and clothing washers. Today, most gray water in the US is commingled with toilet water, and all of it flows through a centralized municipal sewage system for treatment before it gets dispersed back into natural water bodies. But gray water doesn't have to end as sewage. For, you see, gray water is fresh water that's been, so to speak, gently used. Gray water may have mingled with some food from the dishwasher; it could be playing footsy with some dirt, blood, and liquid from the clothing washer, and it most definitely has been in deep conversation with oral bacteria from our bathroom sinks.

That sounds like a lot of dirty play, but it's not. Gray water has great potential for reuse, especially if we consider it an option for irrigating our lawns and plants. Systems for capturing gray water and cleaning it exist and are becoming more common, especially in regions of the world (including the US) where rainfall is sparce and water conservation is a priority. They include a laundry-to-landscape system, which diverts water from your washing machine to your lawn; a branched drain landscape system, which diverts water from your drains (sinks, tubs, showers, and laundry) to your lawn; a shower-to-toilet system, which captures shower water and diverts it to be used in your toilet; and a pumped landscape system, which captures all your gray water in a tank for use on your lawn. Gray water capture is a smart solution to combat water scarcity in dry, drought-stricken areas.

The biggest benefit of graywater systems is that fresh water is left to be consumed by humans. Its secondary benefit is that you can realize cost savings in the form of reduced water bills.

Green Water

The concept of "green" water is fairly new to me. It reminds me of the book written by Doreen Cronin for elementary school–aged children, *Diary of a Worm*. My son Quinn, who's eight years old, loves this book and its companion books, including *Diary of a Spider* and *Diary of a Fly*. *Diary of a Worm* is the story of the day in the life of an everyday worm making his way in the world and, in the process, supporting the health of the earth's soils. The book is both goofy and endearing. It also reminds us that worms have a purpose other than getting stranded after a rain or tortured by little feet squooshing the guts out of them on school sidewalks across the nation.

Green water is food for our soils and plants. It is water absorbed by the roots of living systems. Water that stays in the earth is regenerative for our soils, so green water nurtures our soils and, like worms, supports its healthy functioning.

Black Water

The last water category is a short one. Black water is sewage water. It's water that is highly contaminated, requires treatment, and cannot be reused. It most assuredly is not potable or available for human consumption. Black water carries harmful bacteria and pathogens and always must be commercially treated. Avoid consuming black water. Go with green, blue, and gray!

Sustainable Water Choices

For the Penny-Wiser	• Limit shower time to five minutes. • Shower every other day.
For the Be-Bester	• Install WaterSense toilets, showerheads, and faucets. • "Reuse" water bottle water to make coffee and tea.
For the Bridge Builder	• Plant drought-tolerant grasses, succulents, and bushes. • Avoid laying lawn turf.
For the Nature Lover	• Flush the toilet every other trip. • Install drip irrigation for lawn and deck plants.

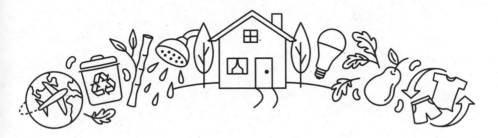

13

· · · · · ·

Trash

I only feel angry when
I see waste. When I see
people throwing away
things that we could use.

MOTHER TERESA

NATURE IS a perfect system of birth, life, death, and renewal. No one thing seems extraneous, and there is an absence of natural "pollution."

If I can claim adherence to any religious tenets, they would be the ones held by Buddhism. I don't believe Buddhism is a religion per se, but a philosophy for living. For me, that is its power.

Buddhist monks describe human life and death in the same language as what occurs in nature. Death in Buddhism is not an end point but a moment of rest in a continuum of living and non-living states. Daisaku Ikeda, the Japanese Buddhist philosopher, describes the human cycle as "repeated cycles of formation, continuance, decline, and disintegration" through which all systems must pass. He goes on to explain how Buddhists perceive human circularity:

> Cycles of life and death can be likened to the alternating periods of sleep and wakefulness. Just as sleep prepares us for the next day's activity, death can be seen as a state in which we rest and replenish ourselves for new life. In this light, death should be acknowledged, along with life, as a blessing to be appreciated.[1]

We see circles and continuity in all things, all cultures. Why not in trash? I may ask, "What was trash before it became so?" The answer: something of value and worth. Why should we see something as having value in one moment and being valueless in the next? I'd ask that we move away from this binary view of things, of materials. If we can zoom out for a moment and see the system of trash with different eyes or through a different lens, we can look anew at what "trash" is and both redefine and rename it.

Trash today is something we don't want anymore. That is not to say someone else doesn't want it. And it is not true that it retains no value. We just perceive it as having no value for ourselves.

Zoom out a little further.

What we perceive as trash at this moment was at some point in the not-too-distant past something we bought or that was gifted, used, enjoyed, and valued for a period of time. At some point, our feelings about the object changed, and we shifted how we valued that object. Inherently, though, the object's intrinsic value did not change.

All things made, all products produced, are made from some type of material or a combination of materials. We are intimately familiar with many of those materials: glass, aluminum, steel, wood, copper, paper, cotton, wool, plastic. Most of these materials are found in nature. Almost all have been transformed in some way to make products that possess features and properties we desire. In many instances, heat is required to transform materials. Some materials need to be pulped and extruded to build a finished product.

Zoom out and relax your eyes.

Materials that come from nature are in and of themselves recyclable. We call them sustainable materials; biodegradable; all-natural. They come from the earth and can go back there. An apple eaten can be thrown on the ground and reabsorbed as a nutrient for the soil. It is reasonable to say that a one hundred percent linen tunic purchased, worn for five seasons, and then determined to no longer be of use *to you* could ostensibly be buried or composted: returned as a nutrient back to the earth.

Of course, we don't bury our old clothing. And very little clothing produced today across the globe is made with one hundred percent all-natural elements. The tunic fabric may be linen, but the thread may be made of nylon and the garment tag of polyester.

Getting Back to Trash

Trash is trash for two reasons. The first is mentioned above: we stop valuing the things we once did and seek to remove them from our lives. The second is a systems challenge: we have developed few post-consumer, post-value mechanisms for things made for human consumption to be processed and returned back to the earth, to be renewed and reborn. Things, and the building blocks of them—materials—die an abrupt death. We know that death as trash.

Materials that go from birth to use to death are living an unnatural cycle. It is a uniquely human construct. One that can be changed. One that must. Today, material trash goes to two places: a landfill (to be buried) or incineration (to be burned). What a waste... of materials!

In the work I do as a corporate sustainability professional, I talk about the value of materials in excruciating detail. Sometimes I feel like a broken record. But valuing and revalorizing materials is my mission and passion. We need to see the path of things and materials as not ending once we are done with them but as a circular system of use, reuse, revalorization, and renewal.

Sorting Is the Solution

Sorting is the biggest systems challenge we face. What we don't value, we don't care about. But we must!

If you ever have an intense desire to comb through the US EPA website on landfill waste to see what materials are finding their way to high-density landfills across the country—I know, such moments fill your days with fantasy—you'd find that some eighty percent of the materials could have been redirected to avoid their fate in landfills. Landfills could be reduced significantly, along with land pollution and methane off-gassing that exacerbates climate change, if we took enough care to sort the materials we use, post-use.

Look, I get it. We're busier than ever juggling our work and household demands, being the emotional center for our kids, and keeping the daily routines flowing, going, and efficiently on schedule as they need to be. By 7 pm, I've already made multiple breakfasts, served up at least two lunches, and am limping to dish clean-up post–family dinner. What often confronts me at the

kitchen sink is a lunch box full of half-eaten items of food, peanut butter–stained and greasy Ziploc bags, and four sets of dinner
dishes and flatware with varying degrees of unwanted, uneaten
heaps of food remnants, waterlogged and begging for a quick
scrape under the faucet and down the disposal.

What about those take-out days, especially during the 2020
pandemic, when restaurant dining became near-obsolete, when
you'd order take-out food for the family and be left contemplating
how to deal with all the various cardboard and paper items, plastic bags, and containers that held your entrees but also various
sauces and vinaigrettes? What goes through your mind at that very
moment? I'll tell you what goes through mine: a momentary sense
of being overwhelmed with managing all of the materials just from
one sole dinner experience.

Yes, sorting can be daunting. I'm not going to deny it. But we
have to internalize a sense of responsibility for managing what
we consume and what we use. We have to know that if we take an
extra three minutes (and let's be real, although it may emotionally
feel like twenty additional minutes to clean up disparate materials
from a dinner take-out, it falls more into the five-minutes-or-less
category) to empty materials of foodstuff, make a quick wash of
it (including those Ziploc bags that can be reused for years!), and
ensure we carefully sort and place items in appropriate curbside
bins for municipal collection, we've done the job of material sorting
well. And no, not all of those containers and bags will be able to go
in your municipal recycling bins. Frustratingly, no.

It's incomprehensible to me why we have so many different
types of plastic. And there are not just seven kinds of plastic. Number 7 plastic alone is an aggregate of so many different types of
plastic and commercially "compostable," biodegradably sus-
pect materials that I find myself shaking my head and wondering,
*Who came up with this labyrinth of materials and byzantine system
of coding?* I'm going to blame ExxonMobil and all the other richly
rewarded, Earth-destroying oil and gas companies that have been
allowed (and government-subsidized for over a century, no less) to

push the burden of responsibility for recycling materials onto the backs of consumers—you and me and the rest of our lot!

So, I get your confusion and understand your anger. We are left to decode what materials can be recycled and those that cannot. The plastic recycling triangles are not easy to decipher, let alone read with the naked eye. And what about those plastics that don't have a recycling triangle imprinted on them? What do you do with those? Something? Nothing? I feel your weariness of having to navigate our patchwork recycling system across fifty states with inadequate recycling laws. We seem to know how to mostly recycle packaging in our home, but how do we recycle well when we are traveling, for work or for holiday? Navigating our post-consumer recycling system within the US is maddeningly opaque.

I ask—often out loud and aggressively to no one in particular while standing in my kitchen or garage—why manufacturers of products can't simplify their packaging for us. Why can't they use a much smaller curated set of materials that they—and we—know are highly recyclable? It would be less work for them, and significantly easier for us, who have to clean and sort and recycle those materials.

We are moving in that direction. We as a nation, and a collective global community, are in the development stages of figuring out how to recycle, downcycle, upcycle, and revalorize materials that are not natural and have no true mechanism for returning to earth to nurture and restore our ecosystem. The hardest materials for us to manage today are plastics, particularly plastics not labeled #1 (PET/PETE) and #2 (HDPE). Take heart. Our recycling systems for hard-to-recycle plastics and other materials, however inadequate today—and they are woefully so—are being developed. Chemical recycling of plastics is an old technology that has gained new relevance and urgency with the climate crisis bearing down on us and the plastic pollution problem growing exponentially. We are at the zygote stage of chemical recycling. The fetus of an idea needs to grow with nurture and care. Chemical recycling for plastics #3 (PVC), #5 (PP), and #6 (PS) are viable but have just recently been birthed. Time and resources are required to develop these babies into hearty young adults who can stand independently and confidently on their own.

Sort: because you care, because you can, and because you are making a difference that will be felt for generations to come.

The Renaming Game

Here's my short schtick, and I'm sticking to it: we need to overhaul how we name "trash" and "waste." We would benefit from retiring those words altogether. We need more descriptive words for the materials that need to have something done to them after we are done using them. They need to go somewhere, but not away and definitely not buried. It should be a goal for all of us to have materials renewed and reimagined. Today's unwanted material doesn't magically disappear, but trash pollution can if we make a concerted effort to sort, recycle, and reuse.

We are making progress in fits and starts across the US in renaming trash and waste. I was pleased in 2018 when I was visiting Boston to see multiple bins for sorting materials post-consumer use at the Verb Hotel, where I booked my stay. Here in Portland, you can find a wall of bins for dropping in materials to be recycled or handled appropriately at restaurants, bars, coffee shops, and grocers.

Instead of trash and waste, what should bins be named? And how many would we need, standing side by side? Here's a list. Some are more obvious than others.

Compost: All food and commercially compostable plates, flatware, and cupware

Recycle: Highly recyclable paper, glass, and aluminum products

Upcycle: All plastics that can be made into high-quality products— #1 and #2

Downcycle: All plastics that can be made into lower-quality plastics— #3 to #6

Hazardous Materials: Batteries, incandescent bulbs, toxic chemicals, and flammable items

Waste-to-Energy: All consumer products that blend plastics #1 to #7 or are #7 only

If we used a more accurate labeling system, people would better understand where materials go and what their next life will likely look like.

Compost: Returned to earth in the form of soil

Recycle: Melted down to be reused again

Upcycle: Revamped to make new products of the same quality as the original

Downcycle: Transformed into new products of lower (but still valuable) quality than the original

Hazardous Materials: Processed responsibly to ensure that chemicals don't find their way into the environment to pollute the land, air, and people

Waste-to-Energy: Hard-to-recycle materials that are man-made and synthetic (e.g., nylons, polyesters, #7 plastics, and cannot-be-disassembled thermoplastics) have no current recycling viability system but can be used to produce energy

Zero Waste

By the cool estimates of the EPA, seventy-five percent of all our trash is recyclable, and between twenty and thirty percent of our household waste is compostable.[2] If we add up those numbers, what do we get? About one hundred percent. That's a zero-waste home right there. But let's just shoot for ninety-five percent and give ourselves some leeway to work toward a trash bin with almost nothing in it. Let's look at the numbers.

Each person in the US generates 4.9 pounds of trash per day.[3] Of that number, a little over a pound and a half of that trash is recycled or composted, which equates to about thirty-one percent of each person's trash being diverted from landfill or incineration. It is informative to see what materials are most likely getting recycled. For the most recent year available (2018), the EPA reports the following recycling rates of common household products:

Home Recycling Rates (by Material)

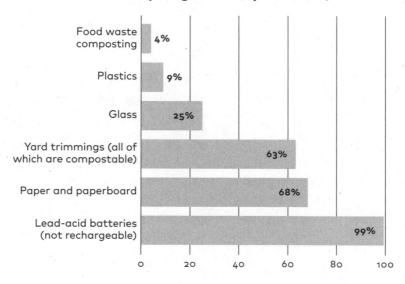

SOURCE: "National Overview: Facts and Figures on Materials, Wastes and Recycling," US Environmental Protection Agency, epa.gov/facts-and-figures -about-materials-waste-and-recycling/national-overview-facts-and-figures -materials.

The good news is we are recycling and composting more items that used to be considered pure waste. Of course, we could be doing better. Paper and cardboard recycling hovers just below seventy percent. Wha? That's easy-town to recycle. Take a look at yard trimmings. All yard "stuff," such as grass, weeds, and branches, is compostable. Along with food composting, if we exert a little bit more effort, our recycling numbers can grow exponentially.

You know what to recycle. Start being more diligent about doing so.

Trust me: a kitchen compost bin is a lifesaver and major trash eliminator (think food scraps and peels, lint, dust balls, paper towels, coffee grinds, tea leaves, and wine corks). A compost bin costs less than $30 and is machine washable. Throw in another $6 for a box of twenty-five compostable baggies and your compost-ing days are set for high gear. For a household of four people, one compostable bag will fill up every one or two days. Over a week-end, when we prep meals for the coming weekday evenings, I can fill up my compost bin a couple of times a day. I'm still amazed at how much "trash" I can avoid by composting my foodstuff. It's an incredible feeling that I want you to experience as well!

Composting can be part of a state's municipal trash pickup, with special composting bins supplied to a home, or it can be installed in the backyard or even developed inside the home. When done right—and it is easy to do—compost soil is ready to be used on out-door plants and lawns after anywhere between two weeks to two months. Composting isn't hard. What is the most difficult hurdle is the initial effort to set up a place and routine and get used to the idea of what goes into the bin. I guarantee you that within the first three weeks of composting, you will be amazed how little goes into your actual trash bin.

Composting pays you in the pocket. Decreasing the size of your home's trash can from a sixty-gallon bin to a twenty-gallon bin, or scheduling trash pickup bi-weekly or monthly instead of weekly, can conservatively save a homeowner at least $10 in trash charges per month, $120 annually. Many municipalities that offer compost bin collection provide incentives for households to compost and whittle down their actual landfill or incineration waste. Check out what your state or municipality has to offer you.

KRISTINA MATTSON

Zero-waste advocate, educator, and community collaborator

KRISTINA MATTSON of St. Paul, Minnesota, is an incredibly inspiring human being. She's a mother of three kids, a former oncology and hematology nurse, and now a stay-at-home mom and zero-waste crusader. After learning through fellow mom friends about where the city's trash went—mostly to incinerators that burned waste and sent pollutants into the air—and how it affects asthma rates in children, she felt she needed to do something where she could. That something was household trash and buildup of residential waste.

Kristina then did something surprising. She read through the UN IPCC's most recent Climate Assessment Report, not an easy read for a layperson. Her conversations with fellow moms, her trust in science, and her internalization as a stakeholder emboldened her confidence that she could take sustainable action and effect meaningful change. She co-founded the organization Zero Waste Saint Paul in 2017 and became a master recycler and composter. The organization's motto is "**A**dvocate. **C**ollaborate. **E**ducate. Together we can A.C.E. Zero Waste!" She's become an active, vocal community builder in St. Paul by working with individuals within her network to understand how they can build sustainability into their lives. She also advocates for sustainable policies at the municipal level, especially in leading the charge to get the city to provide curbside composting. Kristina is no-nonsense yet adamant about the importance she places on sustainability, saying, "You don't have to be an expert. You just have to work to build impact." Kristina makes it clear that she wants sustainability to be accessible to others. She knows it's a process to make behavioral changes. Her approach is, "Let me show you how; let me show you what I do."

Kristina is keenly focused on how and what she purchases, with an eye toward eliminating unnecessary packaging and reducing the trash in her home that comes from consuming. She tries to avoid buying products with any plastic packaging. To help her stay true to that goal, she's moved to conducting most of her grocery shopping at her local grocery co-op, which stocks local and regional products that don't require heavy packaging systems because they've traveled short distances. She shops exclusively with her own reusable bags and brings her own reusable glass containers for transporting fresh veggies and fruits she buys back to her home. And of course, to get to her goal of a zero-waste home, Kristina composts all of her food waste. She also works to collect her neighbors' compostable food waste at a centralized facility—the local church—about a mile away from her house. The unintended consequence of supporting a zero-waste community is the satisfaction she gets from connecting with others in her community.

Kristina has been focused on pursuing sustainability measures for seven years, starting around the birth of her third child. She admits that shopping at the local co-op does cost a little bit more money, but she finds comfort in knowing that the food is locally sourced, non-industrially produced, and so much healthier for her family. She calls it a worthwhile trade-off for eating better-quality food. She's also walking and cooking more because of her sustainable mindset and eating out less often.

Kristina reinforces over and over two big quality-of-life benefits she's received by living more sustainably: greater health and well-being from being more active and eating better, and life satisfaction and personal meaning in supporting others' sustainability journeys.

Sustainable Trash Choices

For the Penny-Wiser	• Shop with your own durable bags (many states are charging $0.05 per bag). • Reuse durable containers for as long as possible.
For the Be-Bester	• Dispose of your hazardous materials responsibly: steel, rubber, treated wood, batteries, bulbs, and air conditioners can all be recycled but need to be taken to special local and state hazmat facilities.
For the Bridge Builder	• Compost all food waste and yard trimmings. • Donate compost soil to local farmers.
For the Nature Lover	• Recycle all glass jars, aluminum cans, jar tops and bottle caps, paper and cardboard, and #1 and #2 plastics. Most people are given this ability through their municipal curbside recycling. • Become a member of burgeoning post-consumer recycling organizations that pick up hard-to-recycle plastics for a fee.

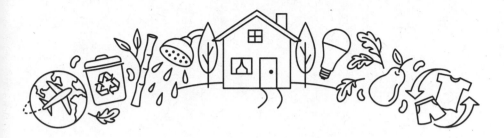

14

. . . . . .

Ownership

Liking is probably the best form of ownership, and ownership the worst form of liking.

JOSÉ SARAMAGO, *The Tale of the Unknown Island*

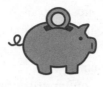

THIS CHAPTER is what you'd call an "outlier" in statistical analytics. Ownership is not an impact category and it's not a framework for matching what you value to sustainability measures you want to pursue. This chapter is really a thought piece to help decipher where your mind settles in valuing the ownership of things. As we get into the heart of the chapter, you'll come to see that the "sharing economy"—renting, leasing, borrowing, reselling, and by-the-hour using of physical things—is correlated with greater personal sustainability, but not in all cases. It's complicated. I'm here to help clarify the good, the bad, and the uncertain as best I can. Keep reading to find out the sustainability "grade" I give to ownership activities most of us have engaged in at some point in our lives.

The Sharing Economy

The sharing economy is transforming entire industries: vacation timeshares, hotels, and errand-running, to name just a few. Equipment rental is succumbing to its demands; rightfully, too.

I'd argue that unless you specialize in a trade or industry, very few of us have need to own non-essential equipment. Of course, if you are a jewelry maker, you will want to own jewelry-making equipment. If you are a landscaper, you will need landscaping equipment. If you are a wood- or metalworker, it makes sense to own the equipment you need to craft wood and metal into furniture.

But the everyday person—no, we don't need (and shouldn't want?) to own equipment. And I am talking about the average, run-of-the-mill home-type equipment we love to hate, like lawn mowers, leaf and snow blowers, and chainsaws.

If you use a piece of equipment infrequently, rent it. If you require equipment for a season, lease it.

I'm even talking about home exercise equipment: bikes, rowers, weights, and climbers. Of course we think we will use them forever, definitely for the next x number of years. We often don't. We tire of them. We move on to another exercise routine. And these hulking machines take up corner space in a lonely room, never to be used again.

Instead of buying them, rent or lease them. Get them off your hands and back to the manufacturers or retailers that are in the business of meeting consumer demand for these products. Have them take your rental off your hands and put it in the arms of the next expectant user.

There are a number of compelling benefits to this arrangement:

- You only pay for the time you use the equipment.

- You are not burdened with managing the sale in the aftermarket.

- Equipment is owned by fewer owners, who retain the equipment's value and responsibility for its longevity.

- Equipment can more easily be refurbished and reused and its material recycled at the end of its life.

- Products and materials can live a circular life and not a linear one that ends with a trip to the landfill, never to return.

Things

Borrowing and handing down clothing, accessories, and shoes is very much an old idea that remains relevant and a very contemporary practice in the twenty-first century. Anyone who's had at least one child birthed into the world knows full well that articles of clothing in the first five years of that (lovely) human's life only get about three months of play before a growth spurt happens and it's back to the ever-revolving purchasing wheel. Most toys have double that lifespan, but they get discarded quickly and voluminously. Borrowing and taking others' hand-me-downs is not only a financially smart practice, but it's also advantageous from a time-resource perspective for parents.

Hand-me-downs and bequeathed items are not just limited to articles of clothing and toy stuff. The best haul I ever received—God bless their souls—was from my paternal grandparents, who passed a month apart from each other, the first on my college graduation day (no joke!). My father and his sister didn't want or need any of their furniture or kitchenware and asked whether I wanted anything. I had just graduated with nothing, literally nothing, to my name. Yes, I wanted things. And I was the recipient of a sectional couch, two sitting chairs in perfect condition (because back then, my grandparents put plastic on everything), several lamps, and a full sixteen-piece dinner set, which I recently saw on sale at an antiques shop in Brattleboro, Vermont, plus flatware. I felt lucky and, even more, grateful.

There's this thing neighborhoods do here in the city of Portland that feels quaint for a medium-sized US city: people paint book boxes, hammer them into the ground, and place a sign on them that says, "Take one, leave one." Community sharing of free books. It's sweet and cool.

Gear

More and more high-profile outdoor gear companies are moving to rent, lease, and exchange models for outdoor hiking, climbing, camping, and water sports gear. Who comes to mind? REI, Patagonia, and Arc'teryx. This sharing "model" isn't necessarily new, right? When you go to the beach, if you aren't a competitive or hobbyist surfer, you rent a surfboard. You do the same for renting jet skis or a catamaran for a day sailing on the ocean. When you go skiing and haven't done so before, you rent your skis, boots, and poles. Why buy something if you aren't sure you'll like the sport or don't see yourself doing it often?

What's different is that manufacturers are employing rental and leasing models for customers who typically walk into their stores to make a personal purchase of their desired gear. Extending rental, lease, and exchange options to individuals is a way to do two things very well:

1   extend the life of existing items that may not get a lot of use from individual customers by themselves; and

2   slow the manufacturing of products, since items that already exist can be used over and over again.

Machinery and Hard Durables

Here, think about those once-a-year or even every-couple-of-years pieces of equipment we may need to use but that sit collecting dust somewhere in our garage or stored deep in the recesses of a jam-packed closet that we're too scared to sort out because it's become a Pandora's box of accumulated things. Why not rent or lease equipment we use infrequently? The Home Depots and Lowe's of the world do just that for individual consumers, facilitating a different kind of sale—a rental and lease sale versus a new one. At do-it-yourself big box retailers or local hardware stores, you can increasingly rent or lease tools like augers, generators, air compressors, and tile saws; equipment for plumbing, drywalling, and demolition; and even machinery like lawn mowers, backhoes, and forklifts. I've heard of some of these pieces of equipment, but I surely have not used most of them myself. You get the picture, though. Rent these babies! No need to buy them anymore.

When it comes to things, clothing, gear, and machinery and equipment, the lease, rent, and exchange model definitely supports a significant increase in one's personal sustainability. Or, looking at the other side of the coin, your carbon footprint will see a reduction if you use these "sharing" mechanisms put in place by retailers. When stuff can live longer, be put to use by more people, and not have to be made new, the emission of greenhouse gases by the manufacturers of these products is dramatically reduced.

Sustainability Grade: A-/B+
By renting things you don't need all the time, you are still consuming "stuff," but you are making a choice to use what is already made.

Resources

Here, I'm particularly thinking about food and water, but the generation—creation and distribution—of renewable energy also applies to this category.

Food

Listen, you know that the outcome of planting a fruit-bearing tree, if we're lucky to have a green enough thumb, is bounty. I remember planting my first tomato plant on the small roof deck of my duplex in Dupont Circle in Washington, DC, back in 1996. I had tomatoes for days. So many tomatoes I gave them away. And that is the very nature of growing your own food. You do it for the curiosity. You do it for the adventure. You may have done it during the pandemic of 2020 because, heck, why not? You were home with plenty of time in a confined physical space, wanting to do something that would get you outside and into nature. But the very act of growing, for whatever reason, has another by-product: sharing. "Here, taste this strawberry. It's ungodly delicious." "Do you like figs? These are awesome. Have them with some honey and feta tonight after dinner." "Are you a salsa lover? These bell peppers and tomatoes paired with cilantro from the herb garden will knock you out. Just you wait!"

Growing fruit-bearing plants, planting a garden, or participating in a community garden in a city defined by limited natural space is beautiful, bountiful, wondrous, and delightful to the senses, but also to our realization that Earth provides when we care to commune with the magic that lays within soils we barely consider as we go about our daily lives.

Water

The same goes for rainwater capture systems. These remain, thankfully, low tech but always effective: a barrel or cistern, either buried or above ground. These "systems" are perfect for urban living. You capture water that falls from the sky, off your roof, and spread that natural love back into the ground by irrigating your lawn, trees, and plants. I know individuals who have multiple water capture barrels on their property for a "just in case" time when they might be needed, say in a natural disaster or during an extreme weather event that overwhelms or disables a septic system. Reuben Deumling (Katherine Deumling's brother, who you'll learn more about in Chapter 16) is one of them. He's a planner. In his worst-case scenario, he says he has enough water to support sixteen of his neighbors for several weeks. Now that's sharing resources.

Energy

I realize that you may not know about or have access to community solar or wind microgrids where you live. These are small-scale energy generation systems for a community's benefit. One way community solar works is by placing solar panels on a church's roof. Church members fund the investment, but they are also the beneficiaries of the energy that is generated, lowering their energy costs over the course of twenty to twenty-five years. It's a distributed energy system that is zero-GHG emitting and that provides a multitude of benefits: clean energy, lower energy costs, and a tighter, more resilient community of individuals with shared interests.

Sustainability Grade: A
If you have taken these measures, you are supporting your own food bounty and helping to conserve natural water resources. Additionally, you are extending your goodwill and health to others in your community who are just as deserving as you. Moving toward the use

of renewable energy is our destiny. Doing so in a democratized way is both human-centric and unifying.

Property
· · · · · · · · · ·

A movement is catching fire across the US: the small living movement. It takes two divergent forms. The first is building, buying, and living in a tiny home. Tiny homes come in various types and sizes. Mobile homes—small homes on wheels—can be as small as eight by sixteen feet (128 square feet) and as large as eight by thirty-six feet (288 square feet). These are cropping up more and more in the fire zone areas of California, allowing residents of the state to move out of harm's way while relying on a place to call "home." Tiny homes, sometimes referred to as compact homes, are permanent dwellings smaller than five hundred square feet. The benefits of owning and living in a small home are manifold and include the following:

- Less energy needed to heat and cool the space
- Less material needed to build the home
- Less land required for the building footprint
- Fewer things to buy to fill the interior of the home
- Significant affordability
- Minimal upkeep

The second form of small living is called an accessory or auxiliary dwelling unit (ADU). These are dwellings that are fabricated on someone else's private property and are either rented out to individuals or families to use or provided as free shelter to individuals without roofs over their heads. ADUs typically are no smaller than ten by twenty feet (two hundred square feet) and no larger than twenty by forty feet (eight hundred square feet).

These small units are attractive to all types and age ranges, from new college graduates and kid-less couples to empty nesters and retirees. ADUs are a particularly innovative solution in high-density areas where housing is often not affordable but there is a great need to provide shelter to vulnerable and marginalized individuals. Accommodating those in need by sharing your private property is a community commons concept and precept of sustainability.

Sustainability Grade: B+

Living lightly on this earth is a desired goal for us all. However, small and mobile homes and ADUs require a material building footprint that has associated GHG emissions. They typically also are hooked into the utility energy grid and, depending on where these homes are located, could still rely on coal and natural gas to heat, cool, and electrify the units.

Mobility (Moving To and Fro)

Bikes and Scooters

Not much needs to be said in this category. Besides walking and running, I consider biking to be one of the more perfect ways to transport yourself to where you need to go. It's quick, breezy, autonomous, and a delightful form of exercise. Ask the Dutch. Or the Danes. They get it and love it. Throw in ebikes, and you are cruising faster, more efficiently, and with less effort, all with zero emissions, to your destination of choice.

Bike-sharing systems within urban environments are the sharing-economy alternative to owning your own bike. The bike hubs have centralized locations in front of grocery stores, by bus stops, and in high-traffic retail districts. Hourly biking rates are inexpensive, and you can leave your bike anywhere once you've decided, "I'm done with pedaling for the day." Bike-sharing systems make biking a no-brainer. The only hurdle you have to overcome is answering the question, "Why not try?"

Scooters are the fun kid activity that's been rejiggered for adults. Although, technically, there are plain old human-powered scooters available for you to use to get yourself to work and back, we all know the increasingly ubiquitous form: the electric city scooter (e-scooter). They seem to be taking over our city streets, with helmetless riders ambling along the roads, commandeering the sidewalks, and leaving their e-scooters flopped down on the ground, a little like a tipped-over human just waiting for someone to pass by and ask to help them up. Nonetheless, e-scooters are a zippy way to get around town and, again, emissions-free. E-scooter systems operate the same way as bike-share systems do: they're easy to join, inexpensive to use, and conveniently located.

Sustainability Grade: A/A-
Bike- and scooter-sharing systems are a great addition to public transportation options but provide more autonomy, freedom, and flexibility.

Vehicle Leasing

To own or not to own, that is the question. Listen, most of us know the advantages and disadvantages of leasing versus owning a car or truck. It depends on its affordability and whether we prefer to upgrade our vehicles as innovations occur in technologies.

This category is pretty cut and dried. If you want to lease a combustion-engine vehicle, sustainability is not high on your list of priorities.

Sustainability Grade: C+/C
If you lease a combustion-engine vehicle, I'll give you the benefit of the doubt that you are leasing so you can pull the trigger faster on moving to a hybrid or electric vehicle when the opportunity comes available.

Perhaps you are thinking of leasing a hybrid or electric vehicle. This is a good decision. Battery life and storage systems are improving at an exponential rate year over year. Leasing an EV makes financial and technological sense and allows you to support vehicle innovations and zero-emitting transportation mechanisms without the worry of having your asset lose most of its value as soon as the ink dries on your contract.

Sustainability Grade: A+

By leasing a hybrid or EV, you are committing to renewable energy transportation systems that help reduce your carbon footprint by some thirty percent of your total, just by this one act.

Ride Sharing

Not good.

I get it. Uber's and Lyft's ride-sharing services have made hailing a ride really easy. It's down to the push of a button, and you can track a little car around your town or city on your mobile phone to know exactly where your ride is and when it will be where you need it to be. And ride sharing is cashless. I mean, who needs money anymore?

But the advent of Uber and Lyft has exploded the number of vehicles on the road. Researchers at the University of Colorado Denver have estimated that total vehicle road miles have increased eighty-four percent due to these new transportation systems.[1] They also acknowledge that more than one-third of us would have not driven somewhere, preferring to walk, bike, or use public transportation, if Uber and Lyft had not been invented.

OK, yes, we can hop in EV cars. But how many times? All of them, or fifty percent of your rides? Likely far less than that. Selecting solely EV rides is not an option currently available, so you have no way of insisting on riding in a zero-emitting car.

And yes, Lyft offsets all of its driving miles by purchasing carbon credits. But this is just a very convenient excuse to keep carbon emitting in support of a business model that is terribly bad for the environment.

Sustainability Grade: D

Ride-sharing services, until they can guarantee that one hundred percent of drivers own or lease electric vehicles, are nearly as bad as the oil and gas companies of the world: profiting from a business model that contributes to worsening climate change.

Is Ownership the End Goal?

A valid question to ask ourselves is whether owning is the end goal we seek. Do we need to own to live a well-lived life, one suffused with meaning, high in the contentment category? Plenty of arguments exist that can validate non-ownership as a liberating, useful, trendsetting, and carbon-reducing endeavor, especially if we view it through a sustainability lens.

Home

Does owning a home have to be the end goal of becoming a responsible adult? Mortgages are for thirty years. And, when we speak about "owning," is it you or the bank that really owns your house? Mortgage payments go to banks. Monthly rental payments go to landlords. Mortgage payments aren't the only cost of owning a home. We pay interest, and a sizable amount, on our long-term home mortgages. Rent payments have no interest attached. Homes require constant maintenance and upkeep, and it falls to the homeowner to employ the needed financial and human resources to complete it. Rental unit upkeep is the sole province of landlords and the property management companies they employ to execute the services. When you own a home, you owe property taxes, unless you live in the handful of states that have none. Renters don't pay property taxes on their rental units.

Perhaps, more to the point, owning a home requires a lot of responsibility, which ties up capital in something that is meant to "be of value" in the future. It also necessarily entails you committing yourself and your resources to that one thing over a significant period of time.

Renting does not have those same types of demands. Renting, arguably, allows us more mobility and a more flexible allocation of our financial and human resources so that we can use them for other endeavors of value to us. Yes, renting is seen as a suboptimal solution to owning a home, but does it really need to carry that legacy baggage?

Can renting a dwelling be seen as a smart sustainability decision? One that allows us to use and occupy pre-existing building infrastructure that is typically located near the amenities we need to live and enjoy life: grocery stores and pharmacies, schools and restaurants, doctors' offices and shopping districts. Can renting be viewed as a way to live less burdened by stuff, giving us the ability to allocate our resources to support sustainable communities, activities, and places?

Vehicle

Most people fully understand and appreciate the value of leasing vehicles. Arguably, you likely fall into one of two camps: either you always buy your vehicle and run it into the ground before purchasing another, or you lease a car for two or three years and then trade it in for an upgraded car with all the new bells and whistles, ad infinitum.

Leasing a vehicle today sure has advantages when you are talking about the electric kind. Battery technology capability is growing by leaps and bounds every year. The size, power, and range of EVs coming out in 2021 would have been almost unheard of when you think about the EVs available in the mid-naughts. They are different machines entirely. And thankfully. With improvements in battery technology comes easier decisions for a greater number of people to justify EVs for long-haul trips, large families, and long daily commutes.

Leasing hybrid and electric vehicles makes darn good sense right now and for the foreseeable future. Dip your toe into this transportation revolution without worrying about resale values and asset depreciation rates. Lease to fall in love.

Clothing

Let's be honest, we feel good when we have an opportunity to buy something new that refreshes our sense of self, whether that be new seasonal colors or the newest trend in pants, sweaters, or jackets. We all need a refresh of sorts as we move through the seasons of the year and new seasons of our life: single, engaged, married, new mom, new job, new town, new decade, new life pivot.

There's been sufficient movement in the rental wardrobe category, catalyzed by the first mover, Rent the Runway. The general model is for individuals to pay a monthly subscription fee and have a select number of "rental" clothing items sent to them to be worn for a thirty-day period. It's a good start to a model that has a long runway (pun intended).

Pamela P., a wealth management investment professional, talks about how she and many of the women in her professional alumni network subscribe to Rent the Runway and all wear the monthly goodies that are sent to them. These include top and bottom accent pieces that brighten and update their owned wardrobes so they don't have to spend time shopping for new items and don't have to purchase and own items they may only want to wear once or twice at most.

Pamela and her friends are onto something big and important. How do we go about taming our clothing consumption desires? One way is to support a diversity of options and freshness of pieces through the use of a rental clothing system. It's really the same concept as in the equipment category:

- We want new concepts that are trendy and fresh.
- We tire of clothing often on an annual, if not seasonal, basis.
- We can indulge our sense of style by renting clothes for limited wear.

By renting clothing available to many, we avoid over-consuming. We also leave the reuse, cleaning, refurbishing, and recycling of that rental clothing to professional businesses within the industry who have the commercial capabilities of doing so in a sustainable and large-scale way.

Toys

Rental models for toys exist, but there's not many currently that have a viable business model. There is Whirli, which allows individuals to create a custom box of toys by desired age range, and Rent That Toy!, which itemizes toys for purchase and prices each with a monthly cost.

The rent-a-toy idea is a brilliant one. Parents know that every four to six months children grow developmentally, if not also physically. For the first twelve years of each kid's life, we get to experience about thirty different versions of that child. And with each new version comes new wants, needs, and desires we seek to fulfill, often around books, toys, games, electronics, crafts, and sports. We buy to entertain or even indulge our children's wants and imaginations. Purchases are made to ensure readiness, advancement, or inclusion with their peers. Needless to say, kids demand and get a lot of toys during their eighteen years under our care. At least once a year (if not more frequently), around a birthday or before a holiday, we as parents pursue the task of wading through closets and drawers stuffed with toys to figure out what's relevant to our children's current developmental period. And then . . . trash time. Or a multi-box drop-off to Goodwill. Right?

Yep, the toy industry is ripe for a successful rental model. Kids don't care about new. They care about experience.

These subscription services need to get away from the consumption-mindset models that they literally box themselves into, though. Most if not all of the material goods subscriptions—shoes, clothes, toys—have consumers pay a monthly fee and allow them to use the products for a thirty-day period. Whirli allows for eight months of use of rented toys, but after that period of time, the toys are said to be the consumer's "forever." That's backward logic. This unstated notion that renting goods is exactly the same as buying goods is an economic fallacy with deeply unsustainable consequences.

The idea behind "renting" goods is to slow the making of new and to prolong and leverage the inherent value of existing products. We should rent what we want and how much we want for as long as we want, so long as we commit to paying the price for those decisions. The accelerated model of consuming rental items—every thirty days—just feeds the same consumption system these rental companies are supposedly trying to modify. Or maybe I fail to understand the sustainability foundation within these models.

What Has Value?

Different people value different things. On the one hand, baby boomers grew up during the economic boom years after World War II. They sought advancement in education and work. They strived to own their own homes, automobiles, and the things—personal possessions—that made "life worth living." On the other hand, millennials are growing up with economic burdens. College tuition is debt-fueled. Owning a home is out of reach. And climate change and its impacts on their lives and livelihoods weighs heavily on their minds. They seek a lighter path to living, one that may mean no children, renting and not owning a home, and sharing goods and services so that their consuming preferences have less of an impact on the environment. The pendulum has swung from one way of living, thinking, and being to its opposite.

So, I ask you to contemplate: Is ownership your preference, or is freedom of experience and a more unshackled existence where your heart resides? Is a lifestyle that places more emphasis on having and consuming things what makes you happy, or does a minimalist lifestyle appeal to you, where you have what you need and not an ounce more?

There is no right answer or way of being. But consider what is the truth in your heart. Whichever way your pendulum swings, personal sustainability is still an attainable reality. Like a pendulum, the weight swings back and forth and is never stuck in one place. And just as you would plot your direction with a compass, determine where you want to go and what measures you want to take to live a more sustainable life. You may decide your first direction is not sufficient, and you may seek to rechart your course.

Our ideas about living and what's important to us are not static but changeable. Knowing our starting point helps us map the direction to our end goal.

part three

GROWING SEEDS

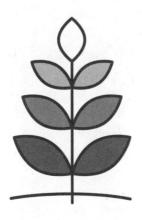

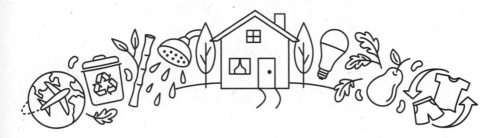

15

......

Curating a Sustainability List

No one can afford to assume
that someone else will solve
their problems. Every individual
has a responsibility... Good
wishes are not sufficient; we
must become actively engaged.

HIS HOLINESS THE DALAI LAMA,
The Path to Tranquility

YOU'VE COME a long way. You've identified what's important to you: your personal value drivers. You know committing to change in your behaviors and decision-making processes is a necessary step toward sustainability. You've learned about the seven impact categories. And you are gathering sustainability measures that are interesting to you and relevant to your life.

There are a few more steps in the process of building a sustainability roadmap. After this chapter, you'll be armed with an action plan built for you, by you.

Creating Sustainability Buckets

An easy way to begin contemplating sustainable actions in our lives is to break down all the options available to us into, say, bite-sized pieces. There is so much we can do in any one area of our life. But, what's reasonable to do? Today, next week, six months from now, and the year after that?

What measures are easy, easy-ish, and effortful? I can tell you I've experienced "analysis paralysis" myself. We think so much about what can be done that we end up doing nothing at all, paralyzed by all the options. Personal sustainability can be overwhelming to pursue. That's why I'm here to simplify your decision-making by breaking down the options available to you into manageable chunks.

You need an approach for how you're going to begin selecting which sustainability measures to pursue. Here's one I recommend:

group sustainability measures into three buckets—small, medium, and large. We can start big, but it's not necessary if you're new to sustainability. The decision to do something, anything, however small, is meaningful. Know and internalize that even small sustainable actions in any one impact category have the ability to effect measurable reductions in our carbon footprints. Sustained effort is the key.

Like most all regimens we pursue—exercising, learning a new sport, eating healthy, reading a book, pursuing an academic degree—we have to keep at our efforts. We don't lose weight by eating one small meal. We don't learn how to ski by taking one lesson. We can't finish a book by reading only one chapter. We are not awarded a diploma after completing one course. Our commitment to the long haul is important. Consistency drives results.

One other thing. Just like when we try to lose weight, we have "bad" days. We cheat. We eat that bowl of ice cream. We have a buttered baguette with our soup. OK, but we don't give up or give in. It's characteristic of the human condition to hit a few stumbling blocks on the road to our goals. When we are pursuing new things, new ideas, new actions, we have moments where our efforts are suboptimal. Shake it off. Be a duck and let the lapse roll off your emotional downy feathers. What's important is that we keep on striving and achieving. For us. For our family. For humanity.

We are ready to categorize personal sustainability measures into buckets of small, medium, and large. This exercise will help you understand which initiatives you feel ready to pursue today and which fall into the "I want to but need more time to contemplate" category.

Small Measures

Small sustainability measures require little to no financial investment from you. They do require modifications in behavior and routine, particularly around how you manage your home tasks and purchasing decisions. Small measures can be implemented efficiently and effectively within a short period of time.

A guiding principle for implementing small sustainability measures is self-awareness: we need to arouse subtle shifts in our perception of what sustainability means, our role in pursuing it, and how our personal buying decisions can and do impact the environment.

In the pursuit of small sustainability actions, you need to commit to a recipe mix of

- forethought;
- a little planning;
- a bit of pre-emptive action; and
- some personal restraint.

EXAMPLE 1: REUSING PLASTIC SANDWICH BAGS

I don't want to continue with a one-and-done practice of using plastic sandwich bags. Instead, I want to reuse plastic bags for as long as they are useful (i.e., they remain intact without holes). Sandwich making and packaging remain the same. When my child's lunch box returns from school, I will compost any remainder of the sandwich and retain the bag for cleaning. I will turn the bag inside out and wash both sides with warm, soapy water. I will rinse the bag of suds and hang the bag to dry overnight. In the morning, I will turn the bag outside in and reuse it for the next day's sandwich prep and packaging. Washing plastic sandwich bags will become part of my nightly dishwashing routine.

EXAMPLE 2: TAKING A FIVE-MINUTE SHOWER

I want to support freshwater conservation and save money on my water bill, too! I don't know how long my showers are typically, but I know they are longer than five minutes. I can set my bathroom fan to five minutes as I enter the shower. I will be conscious of shampooing and conditioning my hair thoroughly but efficiently. While my hair is conditioning, I will lather my body to be cleaned. On the days I need to shave my legs, I will turn off the water to the showerhead, lather each in turn, and shave with the water off. I will turn on the water to rinse off my hair and legs before or at the five-minute mark.

Medium Measures

Medium sustainability actions require both a conscious change of choice by you and a commitment to certain financial investments that will reap dramatic carbon and energy reductions over a short to medium period of time.

For the majority of readers, medium sustainability measures will be in your grasp to achieve.

EXAMPLE 1: BUY LOCAL AND SEASONALLY GROWN FOOD

I care what I put in my body, and I want to support my community and its ecosystem of local farmers. Eating seasonally means just that: you eat only what fruits and vegetables grow during particular seasons of the year. Asparagus, artichokes, and peas in spring. Berries, peaches, mangoes, and melons in the summer. Potatoes, beets, and arugula in the fall. Celeriac, leafy greens, and carrots in the winter. Most grocery stores these days tell you from where each fruit and vegetable is sourced. This "sourced from" information can guide you on how to eat seasonally appropriate food that is fresher and grown closer to home. If produce is coming from North America, it's seasonally appropriate.

Another way to buy locally is to shop for your fresh vegetables and fruits, as well as meats, eggs, and dairy, at farmers markets or to become a member of a community-supported agriculture club. This way of shopping is more expensive but also more immersive, engaging, and, I'd argue, personally rewarding. You literally meet and speak with the individuals and farmers who are selling the food you seek to buy.

For my family of four, my CSA membership delivers a box of fruit and veggies to my door every two weeks on Friday afternoons. I have designated online that my box should be priced at $49. However, I can modify the contents of the box a week before it's delivered. Usually, when I do customize my box, the price tag for the CSA delivery is closer to $90. I typically never need to supplement the two weeks with extra vegetables, but I do the fruits. Almost always, our fruit bowl is nearing empty a day or two before the next CSA box is delivered.

I shop exclusively at farmers markets in the summer and have bi-weekly CSA boxes delivered all year around. My trips to the farmers markets typically cost forty to sixty percent more than if I had bought the same goods at my grocery store. My CSA has a twenty to thirty percent premium on its produce. Is the food fresher? Absolutely, and it lasts far longer than anything I'd buy at my local grocer. Are the fruits and veggies tastier? Yes. Mostly, I notice the difference in the vegetables: they're more vibrant.

The changes in my shopping habits are two-fold. Every Saturday is when I visit my farmers market. It's a ten-minute car ride away from my house. I bring my own reusable bags. I often need cash to make the purchases, and the shopping requires me to walk at least a mile, from booth to booth, to check out what's on offer, converse, and select my goodies. It's well worth the leisurely adventure. My CSA membership requires me to log online a week prior to my delivery and to confirm or modify my box contents. On Friday afternoons, my box is dropped in front of my door, and I need to grab it, unload it, and deconstruct the box for recycling.

EXAMPLE 2: INSTALL HIGH-EFFICIENCY APPLIANCES

To optimize your home's energy use when machine washing and drying dishes and clothes, it's best to install high-efficiency (HE) appliances. A clothing washer and dryer set can be purchased for as low as $1,000, with another couple hundred dollars of outlay to have the appliances delivered and installed. But the investment has a positive payoff or return. Ninety percent of energy used in a clothing washer is for heating the water to clean the clothes. Hot water is not necessarily needed to clean clothes well. By using only the cold-water or eco setting on your clothing and dish washers, you can save $150 per year on your energy bill. Another $5 per year can be saved in water use. By the end of the eighth year of appliances that have an average lifespan of between twelve and fourteen years, your investment has recouped itself and the remaining third to half of the life of the appliances is saving you money year over year.

From a personal systems perspective, having HE appliances, coupled with employing consistently smart practices, makes sustainably practical sense. Run washers only when full. Time dishwashing for every evening and clothing washes for one day every week. Keep the settings fixed so all you have to do is push the start button. Build consistency of practice and habit.

Large Measures

Large sustainability measures really are in a class of their own. These actions reach beyond your wish to reduce just your personal GHG emissions and fossil fuel energy use and move toward the attainment of a lofty, more universal goal: environmental restoration. This higher order of action entails that you consider how every personal decision and action you take will affect the environment and the ecosystem services it provides us, including the quality of the air we breathe, the water we use and drink, and the land we rely on for our personal and pleasure needs.

Large sustainability measures seek to support the notion that you should limit, if not entirely zero out, your personal impact on this earth to the greatest degree possible. Practically, this translates into lowering your personal carbon footprint to levels currently seen in the most sustainable European countries (e.g., Denmark, Sweden, the UK).

In parallel with the goal of reaching a zero-carbon footprint, large sustainability measures seek to help regenerate or lift up the functioning of the earth's systems by restoring polluted land and water systems. Large measures really equate to a two-step dance: fundamentally transforming how you live, consume, and commute, while restoring land, air, and water systems affected by human societies.

More to the point, large sustainability measures require a significant investment of resources both financial and human, dedicated behavioral changes, and a trust in technology that is in a continuous state of advancement. To commit to these I dare say enlightened measures fosters local sustainability in multitudinous ways and deeply cements our commitment to living sustainably, while accelerating a new way of living in symbiosis with our planet.

You should note that not all large measures are available to be implemented in all fifty states. I'm thinking here of using gray water inside the home for toilet flushing. Regulations for its use are determined state by state. You'll have better luck in those states that are water poor, such as Arizona, New Mexico, Texas, and California. So too, the costs associated with some of these measures may be personally prohibitive, like the installation of a geothermal loop system.

EXAMPLE 1: DRIVING AN ELECTRIC VEHICLE

Driving an electric vehicle (EV) is one of the most impactful ways you can reduce your personal carbon emissions. An EV is battery powered, and that battery is rechargeable. Running an EV emits no carbon into the atmosphere. In operation, it's literally a clean machine. An EV doesn't need to be filled with gas—fossil fuels. It lacks an oil-lubricated engine. It is fueled by electricity, which can be one hundred percent from a renewable energy source. EVs are game changers.

They are also expensive. And the battery technology that powers EVs is in a state of rapid transformation. Which means that an EV purchased in 2019 that provides a range of 145 miles will be considered a clunker and not worth the metal it's made of when 2022 EV models hit the market with ranges more than double that amount. What to do?

Option 1: You can purchase an EV knowing full well that battery technologies are changing rapidly but because you want to support this kind of radical transportation transformation. The least expensive EV options for purchase start around $33,000. And then, as they say, the sky's the limit, with luxury EVs reaching into the mid-six figures.

Option 2: You can lease your EV of choice, in look, range, and price. This is both a smart choice and the most affordable one. Leasing an EV allows you to travel emissions-free in a zippy car without concern for the car's aftermarket value. A Nissan Leaf can be leased for around $100 per month. Leasing allows you to get teased into full-blown love of EVs and carbon-free travel.

EXAMPLE 2: INSTALLING A XERISCAPE LAWN

To xeriscape a lawn or property is to both restore a landscape to near-original condition and lay the conditions for local flora and fauna to thrive and maintain resilience in the face of climate change impacts. The elements of xeriscaping include planting trees, bushes, and groundcover that require little water and human maintenance and that are native to the region to foster greater biodiversity and support local pollinators. By employing these design considerations, xeriscape lawns should require little to no chemical fertilizer or pesticide interventions.

Xeriscape lawns are not an inexpensive proposition. I installed one in 2018 on the backslope of the hill behind my home. For an eighth-acre parcel of land, the cost came to just less than $100,000. We installed thirty trees native to the Pacific Northwest, more than double that in low-rise bushes, and hundreds of native groundcover plants. Before any work could be done on the hill, we had to strip the hill of invasive ivy and blackberry vines. This prep work took months. We installed drip irrigation on the hill that is smart controlled throughout the year, and we employ landscapers to come out monthly to weed the hill of fast-growing and entrenched blackberry vines for at least a three-year horizon to ensure the landscaping work and the financial investment of restoring our sloped property to a native habitat would survive and thrive. The upside is that the hill is teeming with wildlife—birds, bunnies, insects, and bees—making a home among the natural beauty of our restored property. This kind of investment beautifies your surroundings, restores the soils and re-covers the land with natives, and provides a welcoming habitat for our non-human neighbors.

IN CREATING these various buckets of sustainability measures, my goal is to lay bare multiple paths forward with a firm grounding of where you find yourself today, where you want to be in the future, and what steps you need to take to get you from here to there.

Personal sustainability is an evolution of learning, trying, modifying, and recommitting to something worthwhile and greater than yourself. The small, medium, large (S-M-L) sustainability bucket approach shows you possible pathways to pursue and a broad spectrum of options to add to your wheelhouse of knowledge. It also allows you to pick a starting point and stake a claim to what is doable for you right now.

Your Sustainable Action Plan

Sustainability will only work if it works for you—it needs to be sustainable in the true sense, over the long haul. Remember Jill Sughrue's overarching message? "Progress over perfection."

I want you to pick and choose the sustainability measures that call out to you in this book. Pursue choices that feel good and right to you. And listen, this book is not a compendium of the universe of sustainability measures individuals can apply in their lives. I've provided groupings of suggestions. Think of them as teasers or an array of appetizers that may satiate you as you begin your sustainability journey, could grow your hunger for bigger and juicier initiatives, or could very well leave you searching for measures that strike to the core of your inner passions. Don't feel limited by the sustainability suggestions in this book. Find intriguing others and make them your own.

To help you build your sustainability list, ponder and then answer the following questions:

- What actions feel reasonable for you to accomplish?

- What measures are you most comfortable taking?

- Which ones do you think you can easily incorporate into your life?

- Which measures seem affordable to you?
  Today:
  In three months:
  By the end of this year:

Remember, there's no need for guilt about the decisions you make. I'm interested in getting your sustainability journey started at this juncture. Any effort you put toward sustainability endeavors is both beneficial and worthwhile. Every sustainability decision, whether large or small, positively contributes to climate change mitigation. The emphasis is on doing.

Here's a list of small, medium, and large sustainability measures grouped by impact category. Remember, this is not an exhaustive list. See them as idea teasers.

Impact Category	Small Measures	Medium Measures	Large Measures
Transportation	Walk to work once a week. Calculate your personal carbon footprint.	Telecommute once a week for work.	Don't take flights for vacations. Buy a hybrid vehicle.
Energy	Designate a renewable energy source from utility. Purchase carbon offsets.	Install an Energy Star HVAC system. Purchase high-efficiency clothing and dish washers.	Install PV solar panels. Replace gas range with electric option.
Home and Property	Install an above-ground rain cistern. Install a smart thermostat for controlling temperature in your home.	Convert hard-scapes to permeable surfaces.	Xeriscape lawn. Install a roof garden.

Impact Category	Small Measures	Medium Measures	Large Measures
Food	Eat only seasonable foods.	Become a CSA member.	Stop eating animal meat.
	Shop local produce.	Grow a garden.	
Material Goods	Shop for clothing less each month.	Buy clothing made from sustainable fibers only.	Don't purchase products with plastic packaging.
	Buy only wool carpets.		Buy only used/ recycled clothing.
Water	Limit the number of toilet flushes.	Install WaterSense faucets.	Install a compost toilet.
	Limit showers to five minutes.	Install drip irrigation in lawn.	Install a graywater reuse system.
Trash	Shop with reusable bags.	Use only durable containers.	Avoid purchasing products that are made with plastics #3, #6, and #7.
	Compost food waste.	Seek out recycling for #4 and #5 plastics.	

Implementing Your Personalized Plan

You've identified your personal drivers, so you know what sustainability measures align with your values.

- Cost savings
- Healthy lifestyle
- Building community and the economy
- Supporting local biodiversity

You know that sustainability measures require you to commit to changes in your behaviors, modifications to how you go about getting stuff done, and an understanding that some financial resources may be required.

You've learned about the seven impact categories that you have control over, either directly or indirectly, to effect change:

1 Transportation
2 Energy
3 Home and property
4 Food
5 Material goods
6 Water
7 Trash

We've grouped a sampling of sustainability measures into the S-M-L buckets related to their size of impact and the personal commitment required to implement.

Now, we need to populate your personal sustainability plan.

The following example worksheet details a sustainability action plan that I might take—a working mom of two kids, married to a professional man, who owns her house and lives in a city with good access to public transportation and biking lanes.

The last two rows of the worksheet ask the following questions:

- What savings or benefits do I expect?
- What actual benefits were realized?

These are important questions. They reference back to the "M" in the SMART goal framework: measurement. The first question is about what you think the benefits will be for you. The second question is an evaluation of the benefits realized. You may want to put a timeframe on when this evaluation occurs: one month, three months, six months, or a year after the sustainability measure was implemented.

Both of the expected and realized benefit questions can be articulated in qualitative terms, quantitative terms, or both. The following are some examples:

Qualitative Statements
- My gut will feel better not eating dairy.

- I expect to lose weight from eating less meat.
- I will get into better shape walking to work and back.

Quantitative Statements

- My family moved from a ninety-five-gallon trash bin to a thirty-five-gallon trash bin by composting our food waste, which saves us $5 per month.

- By using smart irrigation systems to water our lawn, our water bill has been reduced by $10 per month in the summer months.

- By installing an HE dishwasher and clothing washer, we are saving $155 per year on energy and water combined.

Are you ready to get started? Start your sustainability action plan now!

Building a Customized Action Plan

The worksheet to follow lists all seven impact categories and provides space for pursuing one sustainability measure for each. On my website, you will find this and other worksheets you can use to determine your personal drivers, list your sustainability measures according to impact category, plan how and when you will pursue those measures, and check off actions you've completed. Use them all to build your customized action plan, or pick and choose the ones that are most suitable to your organizational style and that will best help you achieve your sustainability goals. For instance, one worksheet allows you to build an in-depth action plan for the sustainability measures you want to pursue within one impact category. Another helps you to aggregate all of the sustainability measures you've committed to pursue daily, weekly, and monthly across all of the impact categories, for easy reference and tracking at your desk or on your refrigerator. You can find and print these worksheets on my website at kategaertner.com.

Step-by-Step Sustainability Action Plan

	Transportation	Energy	Home and Property
Size of Measure	Large	Small	Large
Sustainability Measure	Lease an EV for primary driving	Designate utility to source 100% RE	Install a xeriscape lawn
New Habit Needed? (Behaviors and Processes)	Researched makes and desired preferences Test-drove options Signed lease Need to plug in car 3x/week	Called utility	Researched landscapers Hired landscaper to install Monthly maintenance of weeds
Financial Investment Required?	$400 monthly lease $8 per month in electricity charges	Green utility charge monthly, included in service bill	Yes, $100K $500 monthly maintenance
Benefits Expected? (Qualitative)	Save money Feel great about zero carbon-emitting driving No gas stops to fuel up	Support renewable energy generation	Beautiful lawn Active animal habitat
Actual Benefits Realized? (Qualitative and Quantitative)	Saving money from buying no fuel and no-cost maintenance	Greener grid	Healthy land environment

Food	Material Goods	Water	Trash
Medium	Medium	Medium	Small/Medium
Become a practicing pescatarian	Purchase only all-natural home furniture and soft goods	Install drip irrigation for lawn and deck plants	Compost food waste
Eat sustainably raised fish for protein intake Eat alternative meats and proteins	Researched options Professionally clean furniture and rugs annually	Bi-annual maintenance Turn on and off in spring and fall Manually regulate during prolonged high-heat periods	Investigated local composting options and requested bin and weekly pickup Bought compost bin and bags Scrape all foodstuff into bin Change full bin bag every other day
Not noticeably New meats like Beyond Meat hamburgers have an extra charge of $2.50/hamburger	Sporadic $1,500 in professional carpet cleaning bi-annually	Irrigation cost included in cost of lawn xeriscape Maintenance charge of $500 per annum	$25 for compost bin $8/month municipal composting bin pickup $6/25 compost bags
Weekly meat savings Better digestion Lower cholesterol levels Reduce my personal food emissions	Enjoy the feel of natural fibers Avoid off-gassing from synthetic fibers Longevity of use	More efficient water use Healthier plants	Reduced trash Better disposal of biodegradable foodstuff Support the reduction of landfill methane emissions
Feel great Gut healthy and happy Less lethargic	Buy less Enjoy higher-quality soft goods Longevity of products	Saving 15% on water	25% less trash

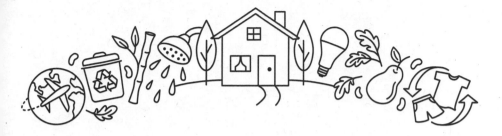

16

......

Finding
Your Voice

Vision without action is useless. But action without vision does not know where to go or why to go there. Vision is absolutely necessary to guide and motivate action.

DONELLA H. MEADOWS, *Beyond the Limits*

AGENCY IS defined by the *Merriam-Webster* dictionary as:

- the capacity, condition, or state of acting or of exerting power.

- a person or thing through which power is exerted or an end is achieved.

You are a person with free will. You have the ability to act on your intention, and through intention you can motivate yourself to take action. Every one of us has the capacity to make change, to effect future outcomes of our own making.

Empowerment is the embodiment of self-determination. We self-actualize that which is important to us. The Buddhist philosophy of life places a strong emphasis on personal responsibility. Buddhist monks speak about the value in living life deliberately. In order to break the cycle of *samsara*—a continuous cycle of being born, experiencing pain and suffering, and dying—we need to awaken our individual consciousness to self-actualization.

I bring up Buddhism not to talk about reincarnation or the meaning of Nirvana but to emphasize the beauty in being the decider of your own fate. You can become who you want to be. You can manifest sustainability in your life. There is no one right way. You make choices, determine strategies, build in adaptations that work for you. You strive. You improve. You fall short and try again. You refine. I want you to remember that you are in control.

What we see, is. What we know, exists. What we do, becomes.

LYNNE SERPE

Empowering sustainable action

LYNNE SERPE embodies personal empowerment in all the best ways. She's a woman who's hit her mid-century with a modern approach to sustainability: make green living "affordable, easy, and convenient." Her vision is to democratize the notion of personal sustainability so that no one feels left out and everyone has a part to play. She states her thinking this way:

> If someone is new to sustainable measures, the fewer hoops one has to go through the better. People are loath to admit they can't afford sustainability or will show discomfort around not knowing a concept or way of doing something. Affordable, easy, and convenient removes any obstacle from people's ability to embrace a green, sustainable lifestyle.

Lynne moved to New Orleans seven years after Hurricane Katrina devastated the city. She was interested in helping to rebuild the Seventh and Eighth wards and, while doing so, fell in love with the people and culture. Her passion is building green knowledge within communities through public library systems. She worked on her Greening Libraries Initiative at Queens Library in New York, a system of sixty-eight libraries, for more than five years. After moving to Louisiana, she re-spun the idea of using public libraries as central hubs for sustainable living knowledge to build an effective system for supporting community composting in New Orleans. The city offered no municipal curbside composting pickup, so Lynne sought to do something about that fact. She began work on creating a composting system for individuals in the community in 2015 at two libraries with a weekly compost pickup at each. By the start of 2020, her community composting system—free to residents and non-revenue-generating for Lynne—had grown to ten sites, collecting over two tons of food scraps each week. Lynne was tired of waiting for someone else, namely the city of New Orleans, to do something about food recycling ("waste diversion"), so she took up the mantle herself. Of course she wanted to push the government to take action, but she also wasn't willing to wait for something she knew she could do herself.

This idea of personal agency and empowerment should be seen as liberating. You can conjure into existence designs that swirl in your head. Don't be stymied by what you think you cannot do. Lynne reinforces the idea that sustainability is about doing what we can, when we can.

Embracing personal responsibility helps you walk the path toward your own personal sustainability. Even if you are someone who has never recycled one thing in your life, today you can decide to do so. One step begets the next. Sustainability is not an all-or-nothing proposition. Life is a process, and so is sustainability.

You decide to be more sustainable. You enact sustainable practices in your life. You see results. You measure. You confirm the worthiness of your sustainable actions. You delve deeper and you embrace sustainability a little more each day. You don't have to live a Herculean life to be a Hercules—an individual hero for the world. Be an advocate—purely through living sustainably—for a sustainable life.

Claiming Yourself as a Stakeholder

What is a stakeholder? It is any individual or entity that can be affected by a course of action. Stakeholders have expressed concerns. In an organizational setting, identifying the key concerns of stakeholders around climate change is a fundamental approach to building an actionable, impactful sustainability plan. A company's obligation is to know who their stakeholders are and to address their concerns in a meaningful and transparent way.

Every one of us is a stakeholder. Stakeholders in life. And stakeholders of sustainability. You may not call yourself a stakeholder. But know you have a strategic role to play in catalyzing positive action around the concerns you have with climate change and extreme weather impacts that are growing from it.

Think of yourself as a strategic actor. The play that is your life and the future lives of your kids is right now. The play's director needs you up on that stage every night, giving your best performance. Your work is important. You're concerned; fearful. You've never been asked to take on such an important role before now. *What if I'm not up to the task?* you think to yourself. You are.

When we hear about global climate change, its scale can be overwhelming. Try not to let it be. Think about the approach behavioral scientists espouse when something is overwhelming. Instead of mentally freezing and becoming incapable of seeing a path forward, they would tell you to chunk up the big thing into smaller, doable workstreams. Make a list. Take and complete one task at a time. Do what you can manage. Tick off the to-dos individually and you'll find you've accomplished the bigger goal.

Being a stakeholder means that you exist, that your concerns are important and deserve to be addressed. The very core of the idea is that you hold a stake in your future and the future well-being of those who are important to you.

Believe in and embody the fundamental notion of stakeholder. Then get going and start living sustainably.

REUBEN DEUMLING

Building agency through discovery

REUBEN DEUMLING is a man who radiates peace and joy, even though he is actively analyzing how to live life as lightly as humanly possible with meaning and impact. He is an intellectual; a student of science. Reuben earned his PhD from Berkeley in energy efficiency and consumption. He's also a husband and a father to a teenage girl. Growing up, he split time between Germany and Oregon. His father maintained forests biodynamically and shaped the sustainability ethic he employs today: preserve the land so it can provide, and be a self-directed agent of change. His mother and brother own the largest plot of privately owned, sustainably managed forest in the state of Oregon. But what he most likes to talk about these days is building a sense of agency among individuals when it comes to sustainability.

Reuben is very clear-eyed when he acknowledges that individuals like to be consoled by the idea that smart men—titans of business or leaders in politics—will solve our climate crisis for the rest of us. Elon Musk will find a way to populate humans on Mars. Jeff Bezos or the founders of Google will invent technology driven by artificial intelligence that will somehow circumvent our growth in physical carbon emissions. We hold out hope for the next "big" thing to solve our seemingly intractable problems, effectively punting work that can be done today further down the road.

Reuben talks about giving people "permission." Permission to pursue sustainability in their lives; to experiment with measures and approaches that feel right and provide satisfaction and momentum for trying more. Give people permission to act and to prioritize sustainability in their lives.

He talks about allowing individuals to "tinker" with what fits with their circumstances and feels right in their lives.

Reuben is focused on having people acquire a sense of agency to pursue sustainability themselves; to give them that experience of doing and knowing what it feels like. He wants individuals to experiment with sustainability and to find out for themselves what can be accomplished that is measurable. This sense of agency in individuals is a bedrock idea for him. He wants people to know that they are in control of what they can implement and accomplish. He also wants to make clear that sustainability does not equate to "freezing in the dark"; that in no small way, personal sustainability and the pursuit of it can be fun, interesting, and rewarding.

Given his academic studies, Reuben focuses on driving his and his family's energy down to ninety percent of what an average American consumes. He calls his energy and water reduction strategy a five-year project that requires very little money spent. His energy reduction plan includes some of the following easy ideas to implement:

- Replace a large refrigerator with a compact one (reduced energy usage by fifty percent).

- Install LED bulbs for all electricity usage.

- Install a "navy shower" valve on his showerhead to stop and start water flow, to conserve water ($2 purchase).

- Turn off the bathroom faucet when brushing teeth.

- Install super-high-efficiency toilets so that bowl flushes consume just 0.8 gallons of water versus the HE flush of 1.6 gallons.

- Employ the toilet-flushing practice of "If it's yellow, let it mellow."

Reuben is also passionate about reducing his material consumption. He smiles when he says he finds meaning in not buying new things. In fact, he finds immense pleasure in learning how the reuse market works, whether that be Craigslist, dumpster diving, or reusing through his social circle. What does he have a keen interest in doing? Not spending money on and not consuming new, virgin resources. His preference is to fix and refurbish things.

Sustainability has improved his life because it's given it meaning. Reuben has three takeaways he'd like to leave you with:

1 You don't need to be an expert to be curious about sustainability in your life.

2 Tackle those measures that seem doable for you today.

3 Give yourself permission to experiment with sustainability. You are not alone. Don't assume there isn't a wide spectrum of people out there pursuing very different paths.

Envisioning

In the summer of 2020, my husband finally convinced me, through the use of months'-long persuasion, to convert our one-car garage into a home gym. I was skeptical, but once the rowing machine, the TRX, and the gym mat were installed, I found myself out there in the non-insulated extension of our home rowing my heart out on a machine with a large TV screen affixed to its front. I hadn't used a rowing machine since my college years. I had remembered not enjoying it much. But the TRX and dumbbells weren't raising any mental motivation endorphins in my head.

This is how I found myself rowing on a stationary machine down a virtual Kafue River, a tributary of the Zambezi River in Zambia. My guide, Steve O., was a former British rowing Olympian turned competitive triathlete and rowing coach to Zambian middle schoolers, as well as my companion to guide my rowing efforts up and down the banks of this African paradise. Steve O. was not just my guide, he was my personal trainer, rowing coach, and local historian, teaching me equally about how to perfect my rowing stroke as well as giving me the history of Zambia, and more broadly Africa, and the importance of the Kafue River to the livelihoods of those who live in the six countries through which it flows: Angola, Zambia, Namibia, Botswana, Zimbabwe, and Mozambique.

I did not have to imagine what the Kafue River looked like; I was on it. I had a soul's-eye perspective sitting just above and in front of Steve O.'s head, where I could view his strapped-in feet and the rhythmic movement of his arms as he rowed his way down the waterway. I was able to experience the thrill of elephants wading into the river and the threat of hippopotamuses raising their heads above water beyond the immediate banks to view the rowing intruders. I was given a map of our rowing course for each session. And wonderfully, I was a teammate and rowing partner of Steve O.'s through seventeen planned sessions that started easy, grew in intensity and length, and measured my improvements in strength and power throughout the entire exercise regimen.

My initial skepticism melted into admiration. Here was a form of exercise I had failed to appreciate for more than twenty-five years, avoided without regret, and came to embrace quickly and definitively because of the way it weaved a story, an experience for me, that was compelling and meaningful. I could leave the mental confines of my home and row in Africa among the wildlife and expansive beauty of the Kafue River while getting into physical shape and seeing that progress through tracked measurements of my stamina, strength, and longevity. Brilliant.

The value of measurement and goal setting to meet with success. The power to envision the seventeenth session at the start of the first and, through incremental steps, ongoing commitment, and personal application, get to the end.

Mental Mapping

You can apply the same methodology for envisioning your sustainable future through the following steps:

- Knowing where you are going

- Determining what the end goal looks like

- Mapping the path from start to end and all the steps to get there

- Pacing yourself—reaching stretch goals takes time, commitment, and perseverance

- Enjoying the journey through a sense of curiosity, continuous learning, and an open heart

- Pairing up with a partner, someone of like mind and constitution, to share the experience

- Measuring progress made toward your end goal

- Flowing in the moment, and trusting the process of doing

- Celebrating your accomplishments

If you can envision yourself doing something, you are more likely to make the outcome happen. Try to envision the sustainable future you want for yourself and then map the journey.

Dr. Gail Matthews, a clinical psychologist from Dominican University of California, studied what actions taken by individuals reinforced the realization of meeting articulated goals.[1] She found that individuals were thirty-three percent more successful at accomplishing their desired goals if they performed the following:

1 Stated their goals
2 Wrote their goals down
3 Rated the level of difficulty in achieving the goals
4 Wrote a list of actions needed to accomplish them
5 Shared their goals with others
6 Provided weekly updates on progress made in reaching their goals

Of the individuals who merely stated their goals, forty-three percent of them met with success. Of the individuals who performed all six of the above tasks, more than three-quarters reached the goals they set out for themselves. Envisioning your future sustainable self and reinforcing those goals with an action plan will actualize that vision.

So, what are you waiting for? Download the sustainability worksheets described in the previous chapter and get your creative juices flowing. You know exactly the sustainability measures you want to pursue. Start filling in the steps you need to get there. Fire up your printer and post your sustainability goals on your refrigerator or your home office whiteboard. Keep them prominently displayed, and don't be scared to get them "dirty": mark them up so you can see your progress, successes, and the challenges encountered.

Your sustainability action plan? It's a living document. A work in progress. And remember, as with most non-competitive goals, much of the personal reward comes from submitting to the process. We learn (and grow) through doing. We are enriched by the very experience we have decided to submit ourselves to. Enjoy the journey!

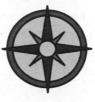

Conclusion
Being a Lodestar

A LODESTAR is defined by *Merriam-Webster* as:

- a star that leads or guides.
- one that serves as an inspiration, model, or guide.

A funny thing happens when you strive for what you believe in: you get noticed. When you fight for what's considered a universal right, there is might to your efforts. Success is not about winning. Often, it is more about the process of trying, failing, and not giving up on ideas you value.

Systems—economies, policies, practices, social norms—are built over decades and centuries. They are designed by human beings. They don't turn on a dime. But systems can change by a chipping away of beliefs, practices, and norms that no longer serve a collective good. Building sustainability into your life is a new way of living. It's a new system of operating. It's turning a ship seventy degrees to the right. It requires some consideration, coordination, and time.

I have a story of hope to tell you. It's a story of kids; our future. It's a story of environmental harm, social justice, and universal human rights we "hold to be self-evident." It's an American story. It's a story of risk and daring, of improbability and revelation, and of acknowledgment and movement toward a sustainable world. It is also a story of failure. Take heart. This story has not reached its ending, although its first chapter has ended. It's a good story. Let me tell you it now.

The story is about a court case filed back in 2015 during the Obama administration. Its name is *Juliana v. United States*. It originated in southern Oregon, but its aim was the whole of America. It involves twenty-one kids—or I should say, more specifically, the lawsuit was filed by them, who were at the time all under the age of twenty; a group of Generation Z individuals. The kids hailed from ten states from various regions across the US, including Alaska and Hawaii. They were picked for their representation of America: white, Black, Native American, Asian; male and female; straight and LGBTQ+.

The lawsuit was a simple one in spirit. The twenty-one kids, with Kelsey Juliana as the lead plaintiff, were asking the federal government to quit its reliance on fossil fuels. Juliana et al.'s argument was that the use of fossil fuels is "causing climate change, endangering their future, and violating their constitutional rights to life, liberty, and property."[1]

In an interview with Steve Kroft, Juliana is asked how important this lawsuit is to her. She replies, "This case is everything ... We have everything to lose if we don't act on climate change right now, my generation and all the generations to come."[2] In late October 2020, after five years of winding its way through the Oregon Supreme Court with the Trump administration's Justice Department providing counterarguments to dismiss the case, the Oregon Supreme Court struck it down based on the scope of the "public trust doctrine" as it exists today.

Without getting too into the weeds on the exact reasons for dismissing the case, Oregon's Supreme Court stated the following in its decision:

> We hold that the public trust doctrine *currently encompasses* navigable waters and the submerged and submersible lands underlying those waters. Although the public trust is *capable of expanding* to include more natural resources, we do not extend the doctrine to encompass other natural resources at this time.[3]

In the five years of lawsuit wrangling, several revealing admissions were uncovered, the first from the federal government itself. Julia Olson, the defendants' lawyer, constructed a historical timeline back to the first federal administration briefed on the reality that burning fossil fuels causes climate change. The timeline goes back fifty years to the presidency of Lyndon Johnson. Olson told Kroft that the government admits—does not deny—that fossil fuels cause climate change. So too,

> [The federal government] does not dispute that we are in a danger zone on climate change. And they don't dispute that climate change is a national security threat and a threat to our economy and a threat to people's lives and safety. They do not dispute any of those facts of the case.[4]

A year into the lawsuit's filing, an Oregon federal judge, Ann Aiken, wrote in her decision not to dismiss the case, "Exercising my reasoned judgment, I have no doubt that the right to a climate system capable of sustaining human life is fundamental to a free and ordered society."[5]

This case, *Juliana v. United States*, is timely. Its concerns are so relevant to your daily life. And it failed in its mission. But it was not a failure.

It exposed the federal government's omissions of knowledge about climate change and its complacency to take measures to mitigate the source of global warming. The lawsuit uncovered the court's sentiment that individuals have a constitutional right to a stable climate. And the lawsuit set a precedent of sorts. In the words of the Oregon Chief Justice Martha Walters in her dissenting opinion, "The court explicitly left the door open for future claims related to public trust resources and the state's duty to protect them." She also made an appeal to us all:

> The time is now. Our forests, our waters, and our children cannot wait.[6]

The message I'd like you to internalize is that climate change mitigation through your sustainable actions is a cause worth pursuing. Sustainability is our "now" topic. It is timely. It is important. It is meaningful.

I want you to make personal sustainability your lodestar: your personal mission, your fixed point to guide you. Make sustainability your destination.

Be the showcase example of hope and promise, fortitude and strength, joy and lightness to your kids. They look up to you and seek to follow in your footsteps. Be their compass to a more sustainable world. It's in your grasp. You just have to reach for it and then, with deep faith and abundant confidence, make the leap to a lifestyle worth living.

We have to be all-in in support of personal change-making. This book does not ask the same level of sustainability from every person who reads it nor from every individual alive. This sustainability book is about acknowledging that climate change is real and that it is already negatively affecting our lives and livelihoods in ways large and small.

I hope this book has shown you your ability to build sustainability into your life. You are able. You can, in no small measure, effect change and make sustainability a priority, a way of life, habit-forming, and the norm: for yourself, your family, and your community. This is no exaggeration: personal sustainability is your destiny.

Acknowledgments

I HAVE SO many to thank in getting this book to publication, and inevitably I will fail to acknowledge someone who was instrumental. Please forgive me for any oversight that may occur. It was not intentional. Jim Newcomer, thank you for believing in me and being my first confidant and ongoing fan. Amy Hall-Bailey, thank you for being a believer, a partner, and the person who brought my ideas to life visually, appealingly so.

To Patraic Reagan: you are my best friend, my big love, and my rock, who keeps me uplifted and rallies me during my low moments, which are plentiful. This book absolutely would not be a living, physical thing without your belief in me.

I give thank-yous to many friends who helped me throughout this process, including Susy Struble, Melody Jones, Melanie Bowen, Pamela Southerling, Chris Mahdik, Katherine Deumling, and Renee Shade. I send a shout-out to those who pointed me to individuals who live, breathe, and do sustainability in their lives every single day: those I profile in the book. I want to thank my Reagan family, who are always joyful and filled with goodness and who support me in everything I do. I want to acknowledge Peggy Buege especially. She became my book avatar, unwittingly. Peggy, your voice, perspective, thoughts, and recommendations guided me along the way, chapter by chapter, to make this book as accessible as it needs to be for readers like you. I love you, Holly Silas, for being my eldest sister, best friend, and steadiest confidante. Love, you, Marion, Caroline, and Janey Silas. I adore you three like my own daughters. Thank you for weighing in on this book. Lastly, I give a shout-out to my dad, who remains excited to read my book.

I want to acknowledge a deep well of gratitude to my adopted Page Two family, including Jesse Finkelstein, Amanda Lewis, Caela Moffet, Peter Cocking, Taysia Louie, Elana Dublanko, Meghan O'Neill, Lorraine Toor, and the rest of the brilliant team that helped me conceptualize this book and refine my thoughts and the message within; edited my words fiercely; kindly, gently, but firmly kept me on track and moving forward; and were there alongside me to birth my first literary baby. Thank you! I send out a special thanks to Jenny Govier, my great copyeditor, who most definitely made my book better, clearer, more concise, and snappier.

I "fell in love" with Donella H. Meadows' mind, clarity of thought, and understanding of systems after reading her primer on systems, *Leverage Points: Places to Intervene in a System*. Then my heart fell when I realized that she had been a professor during my time as an undergraduate student at Dartmouth College and I hadn't known it. I missed my chance to bask in her brilliance when I was a young student not yet aware of how important the study of environmental science would become in my life. Donella is my intellectual lodestar. If you find yourself curious about her writings, read *Leverage Points*. Not only does she make the complex ideas easy to understand, but she bridges science, economics, politics, religion and spirituality into an overriding philosophy of living, muddling along, and persevering.

Notes

Chapter 1: Sustainability: An Old Idea with Renewed Relevance

1 "Great Depression History," History.com, history.com/topics/great
   -depression/great-depression-history.
2 Jake Nevins, "The Imperative of Personal Sacrifice, Today and during World
   War II," *New York Times Magazine*, April 3, 2020, nytimes.com/2020/04/03/
   magazine/personal-sacrifice-coronavirus-world-war-ii.html.
3 Stats in this section cited in Laura Parker, "Fast Facts about Plastic Pollution,"
   National Geographic, December 20, 2018, nationalgeographic.com/science/
   article/plastics-facts-infographics-ocean-pollution.
4 John R. Ehrenfeld, "Sustainability Redefined: Setting a Goal of a Flourishing
   World," MIT *Sloan Management Review*, February 6, 2014, sloanreview.mit
   .edu/article/sustainability-redefined-setting-a-goal-of-a-flourishing-world.
5 Ibid.

Chapter 3: Committing to Change

1 Jacquelyn Cafasso, "How Many Cells Are in the Body? Fast Facts," Health
   line.com, July 18, 2018, healthline.com/health/number-of-cells-in-body.

Chapter 4: Getting Curious about Carbon

1 2016 figure from "CO_2 Emissions," World Bank, data.worldbank.org/
   indicator/EN.ATM.CO2E.PC.
2 The US EPA defines a typical passenger vehicle to be one with a real fuel
   economy of 21.6 miles, driven approximately 11,400 miles annually.
   "Greenhouse Gas Emissions from a Typical Passenger Vehicle," Office of
   Transportation and Air Quality, US Environmental Protection Agency, May
   2014, nepis.epa.gov/Exe/ZyPURL.cgi?Dockey=P100JPPH.txt.
3 2019 figures from World Data Atlas, Knoema, knoema.com/atlas, except for
   that of France, which is the 2014 figure from "CO_2 Emissions," World Bank,
   data.worldbank.org/indicator/EN.ATM.CO2E.PC.
4 "New UNICEF Report Ranks Children's Well-Being in 29 of World's Richest
   Countries," UN News, April 10, 2013, news.un.org/en/story/2013/04/
   436712-new-unicef-report-ranks-childrens-well-being-29-worlds-richest
   -countries.

5 "United Kingdom—CO_2 Emissions Per Capita," World Data Atlas, Knoema, knoema.com/atlas/United-Kingdom/topics/Environment/CO2-Emissions -from-Fossil-fuel/CO2-emissions-per-capita.

Chapter 5: Bias to Action

1 Steve Kroft, "The Isle of Eigg," *60 Minutes*, CBS News, June 24, 2018, cbsnews.com/news/60-minutes-the-isle-of-eigg.

Chapter 6: Living Lightly, Living Well

1 "Animal Pollination," U.S. Forest Service, USDA, fs.fed.us/wildflowers/ pollinators/animals/index.shtml.

Chapter 7: Transportation

1 UN Intergovernmental Panel on Climate Change, *Special Report: Global Warming of 1.5°C* (Geneva: World Meteorological Organization, 2018), ipcc.ch/sr15.
2 Jil McIntosh, "How It Works: Regenerative Braking," Driving, October 9, 2019, driving.ca/column/how-it-works/how-it-works-regenerative-braking.
3 US Department of Health and Human Services, *Physical Activity Guidelines for Americans*, 2nd ed. (Washington, DC: US Department of Health and Human Services; 2018), health.gov/sites/default/files/2019-09/Physical_ Activity_Guidelines_2nd_edition.pdf, 28.
4 American Society of Civil Engineers, *2017 Infrastructure Report Card: A Comprehensive Assessment of America's Infrastructure* (Reston, VA: American Society of Civil Engineers, 2017), infrastructurereportcard.org/wp-content/ uploads/2016/10/2017-Infrastructure-Report-Card.pdf, 77.
5 Ibid., 76.

Chapter 8: Energy

1 "Safer Storage of Spent Nuclear Fuel," Union of Concerned Scientists, March 24, 2011, ucsusa.org/resources/safer-storage-spent-nuclear-fuel.
2 "How Many Nuclear Power Plants Are in the United States, and Where Are They Located?" US Energy Information Administration, FAQs, last updated May 3, 2021, eia.gov/tools/faqs/faq.php?id=207&t=3.
3 David Biello, "Spent Nuclear Fuel: A Trash Heap Deadly for 250,000 Years or a Renewable Energy Source?" *Scientific American*, January 28, 2009, scientificamerican.com/article/nuclear-waste-lethal-trash-or-renewable -energy-source.

Chapter 9: Home and Property

1 Amy Tikkanen, "Hearst Castle," *Encyclopedia Britannica*, britannica.com/
place/La-Casa-Grande; Mark J. Perry, "New US Homes Today Are 1,000
Square Feet Larger Than in 1973 and Living Space per Person Has Nearly
Doubled," AEIdeas (blog), American Enterprise Institute, June 5, 2016,
aei.org/carpe-diem/new-us-homes-today-are-1000-square-feet-larger
-than-in-1973-and-living-space-per-person-has-nearly-doubled.

2 Sheri Koones, "Why Millennials Are Buying Smaller, More Efficient Houses,"
Forbes, October 18, 2019, forbes.com/sites/sherikoones/2019/10/18/why
-millennials-are-buying-smaller-more-efficient-houses.

3 "U.S. Cities Factsheet," Center for Sustainable Systems, University of
Michigan, Pub. No. CSS09-06, 2020, css.umich.edu/factsheets/us-cities
-factsheet.

4 John G. Waite and Margot Gayle, "Preservation Brief 27: The Maintenance
and Repair of Architectural Cast Iron," New York City Landmarks
Preservation Commission and National Park Service, October 1991, nps
.gov/TPS/HOW-TO-PRESERVE/briefs/27-cast-iron.htm.

5 "Manhattan, NY Rental Market Trends," RentCafé, accessed in 2018, rent
cafe.com/average-rent-market-trends/us/ny/Manhattan; "San Francisco,
CA Rental Market Trends," RentCafé, accessed in 2018, rentcafe.com/
average-rent-market-trends/us/ca/san-francisco/; "Chicago, IL Rental
Market Trends," RentCafé, accessed in 2018, rentcafe.com/average-rent
-market-trends/us/il/Chicago.

6 "Average Number of People per Household in the United States from 1960
to 2020," Statista, accessed June 2021, statista.com/statistics/183648/
average-size-of-households-in-the-us.

7 Maura McCarthy, "Rethink, Recycle, Rebuild: How Deconstructing a Home
Makes Environmental and Economic Sense," *HuffPost*, December 6, 2017,
huffpost.com/entry/rethink-recycle-rebuild-h_b_3861930.

8 As cited in EarthTalk, "How Fertilizers Harm Earth More Than Help Your
Lawn," *Scientific American*, July 20, 2009, scientificamerican.com/article/
how-fertilizers-harm-earth.

9 Ibid.

10 Maureen Gilmer, "5 Fundamentals of Xeriscape," Landscaping Network,
landscapingnetwork.com/landscape-design/xeriscape.html.

11 Kristen Hicks, "Xeriscaping: How to Make a Drought-Tolerant Landscape,"
Expertise.com, updated May 5, 2021, expertise.com/landscaping/
xeriscaping-drought-tolerant-landscaping.

12 "Bioswales," Natural Resources Conservation Service, US Department of
Agriculture, nrcs.usda.gov/wps/portal/nrcs/detail//?cid=nrcs142p2_008505.

Chapter 10: Food

1   "Oregon Agriculture," *Farm Flavor*, farmflavor.com/oregon-agriculture.

2   "Community Supported Agriculture," LocalHarvest, localharvest.org/csa/.

3   Kris Gunnars, "Protein Intake: How Much Protein Should You Eat per Day?" Healthline, October 1, 2020, healthline.com/nutrition/how-much-protein -per-day.

4   You can find out more about protein-rich foods, our daily requirements, and the protein amounts that non-meat sources provide on the USDA's MyPlate website at myplate.gov/eat-healthy/protein-foods.

5   Alastair Bland, "Is the Livestock Industry Destroying the Planet?" *Smithsonian Magazine*, August 1, 2012, smithsonianmag.com/travel/ is-the-livestock-industry-destroying-the-planet-11308007.

6   Ibid.

7   John Vidal, "10 Ways Vegetarianism Can Help Save the Planet," *The Guardian*, July 18, 2010, theguardian.com/lifeandstyle/2010/jul/18/ vegetarianism-save-planet-environment.

8   Ibid.

9   Justin Worland, "How a Vegetarian Diet Could Help Save the Planet," *Time*, March 21, 2016, time.com/4266874/vegetarian-diet-climate-change.

10 Bahar Gholipour, "Lab-Grown Meat May Save a Lot More Than Farm Animals' Lives," NBC News MACH, April 6, 2017, nbcnews.com/mach/ innovation/lab-grown-meat-may-save-lot-more-farm-animals-lives -n743091.

11 Corby Kummer, "The Problem with Fake Meat," MIT *Technology Review*, March 31, 2015, technologyreview.com/2015/03/31/168452/the-problem -with-fake-meat.

12 Federation of American Societies for Experimental Biology, "Quantifying the Environmental Benefits of Skipping the Meat," *ScienceDaily*, April 4, 2016, sciencedaily.com/releases/2016/04/160404170427.htm.

13 Ginger Hultin, "Lab-Grown Meat: Exploring Potential Benefits and Challenges of Cellular Agriculture," *Food & Nutrition*, February 27, 2017, foodandnutrition.org/march-april-2017/lab-grown-meat-exploring -potential-benefits-challenges-cellular-agriculture.

14 Ibid.

15 Ibid.

16 "Report Highlights Growing Role of Fish in Feeding the World," Food and Agriculture Organization of the United Nations, May 19, 2014, fao.org/ news/story/en/item/231522.

17 Marc Gunther, "Can Deepwater Aquaculture Avoid the Pitfalls of Coastal Fish Farms?" *Yale Environment 360*, January 25, 2018, e360.yale.edu/ features/can-deepwater-aquaculture-avoid-the-pitfalls-of-coastal-fish -farms.

18 Ibid.

19 As cited in ibid.

Chapter 11: Material Goods

1   There are fifteen types of natural fibers that are sourced from plants and animals (which include arachnids, oh my!). The Food and Agriculture Organization of the United Nations provides information on all of them at fao.org/natural-fibres-2009/about/15-natural-fibres/en.

2   "History of Jeans and Denim," historyofjeans.com.

3   "Service," Denham (website), denhamthejeanmaker.com/en/about/service -co.html.

4   Julian M. Allwood et al., *Well Dressed? The Present and Future Sustainability of Clothing and Textiles in the United Kingdom* (Cambridge: University of Cambridge Institute for Manufacturing, 2006), researchgate.net/ publication/282249347_Well_Dressed_The_Present_and_Future_ Sustainability_of_Clothing_and_Textiles_in_the_United_Kingdom, 2.

5   "Global Synthetic Fibers Industry Factsheet 2020: Top 10 Synthetic Fiber Manufacturers in the World," *BizVibe*, June 23, 2020, blog.bizvibe.com/ blog/textiles-and-garments/top-10-synthetic-fiber-manufacturers.

6   Alexandra Alter, "Yet Another 'Footprint' to Worry About: Water," *Wall Street Journal*, February 17, 2009, wsj.com/articles/SB123483638138 996305.

7   Elisa Tonda, head of the Consumption and Production Unit at the UN Environment Programme, as cited in "UN Launches Drive to Highlight Environmental Cost of Staying Fashionable," UN News, March 25, 2019, news.un.org/en/story/2019/03/1035161.

8   Andrew Barber and Glenys Pellow, "LCA: New Zealand Merino Wool Total Energy Use," 5th Australian Life Cycle Assessment Society (ALCAS) Conference, Melbourne (2006), citeseerx.ist.psu.edu/viewdoc/download? doi=10.1.1.553.6556&rep=rep1&type=pdf, 8.

9   Nicholas Gilmore, "Ready-to-Waste: America's Clothing Crisis," *Saturday Evening Post*, January 16, 2018, saturdayeveningpost.com/2018/01/ready -waste-americas-clothing-crisis.

10 Ibid.

11 Anna De Souza, "This Is What Really Happens to Your Used Clothing Donations," *Reader's Digest*, February 26, 2020, rd.com/article/what -happens-used-clothing-donations.

12 Gilmore, "Ready-to-Waste."

Chapter 12: Water

1   Three percent of all water found on Earth is potable (drinkable), but of that number, only 1.2 percent is readily available for human consumption; the other 1.8 percent is locked up in glaciers and icefields.

2   "Water Scarcity," World Wildlife Fund, worldwildlife.org/threats/water-scarcity.

3   Gregg Semler, CEO of InPipe Energy, in video discussion with the author, February 2021.

4   For a high-efficiency toilet, between one and two gallons of water are used per flush. See "Toilet," Water Footprint Calculator, watercalculator.org/posts/toilet/.

5   Aryn Baker, "Cape Town Is 90 Days Away from Running Out of Water," *Time*, January 15, 2018, time.com/5103259/cape-town-water-crisis, emphasis added.

Chapter 13: Trash

1   Daisaku Ikeda, "Mahayana Buddhism and Twenty-First Century Civilization," lecture at Harvard University, Cambridge, MA, September 24, 1993, daisakuikeda.org/sub/resources/works/lect/lect-04.html.

2   During the last few years, much data was removed from the EPA website, including this recycling figure, but other sites have retained the information, such as these sources: Drew Brucker, "50 Recycling and Landfill Facts That Will Make You Think Twice about Your Trash," Rubicon Blog, November 14, 2018, rubicon.com/blog/statistics-trash-recycling; "11 Facts about Recycling," DoSomething.org, dosomething.org/us/facts/11-facts-about-recycling#fn3. Figures on compostable waste are from "Composting at Home," US Environmental Protection Agency, epa.gov/recycle/composting-home.

3   "National Overview: Facts and Figures on Materials, Wastes and Recycling," US Environmental Protection Agency, epa.gov/facts-and-figures-about-materials-waste-and-recycling/national-overview-facts-and-figures-materials.

Chapter 14: Ownership

1   Alejandro Henao and Wesley E. Marshall, "The Impact of Ride-Hailing on Vehicle Miles Traveled," *Transportation* 46 (2019), doi.org/10.1007/s11116-018-9923-2.

Chapter 16: Finding Your Voice

1   Gail Matthews, "The Impact of Commitment, Accountability, and Written Goals on Goal Achievement," presentation, 87th Convention of the Western Psychological Association, Vancouver, BC, 2007, scholar.dominican.edu/psychology-faculty-conference-presentations/3.

Conclusion: Being a Lodestar

1   Steve Kroft, "The Climate Change Lawsuit That Could Stop the US Government from Supporting Fossil Fuels," *60 Minutes*, CBS News, June 23, 2019, cbsnews.com/news/juliana-versus-united-states-climate-change -lawsuit-60-minutes-2019-06-23.

2   Ibid.

3   Pete Danko, "Oregon High Court Rejects Youth Bid to Force Action on Climate Change," *Portland Business Journal*, October 22, 2020, bizjournals .com/portland/news/2020/10/22/oregon-supreme-court-rules-against .html, emphasis added.

4   Kroft, "The Climate Change Lawsuit."

5   Ibid.

6   Martin Macias Jr., "Oregon Supreme Court Affirms Dismissal of Climate Change Lawsuit," *Courthouse News Service*, October 22, 2020, courthouse news.com/oregon-supreme-court-affirms-dismissal-of-climate-change -lawsuit/.

Additional Resources

Understand the challenges of improving efficiency through the **Jevons Paradox** by reading "The Efficiency Dilemma" by David Owens in the *New Yorker*: newyorker.com/magazine/2010/12/20/the-efficiency-dilemma.

Find out if your organization is a member of **B Lab**: bcorporation.net/about-b-lab.

Learn about the **Academy for Systems Change** through the Donella Meadows Project: donellameadows.org.

Read more about the **"Three Sisters" crops** in Robin Wall Kimmerer's *Braiding Sweetgrass: Indigenous Wisdom, Scientific Knowledge, and the Teachings of Plants* (Milkweed Editions, 2013).

Learn about **Otto Scharmer's Theory U framework** for change through the Presencing Institute: presencing.org.

If you're ready for a wake-up call, read the **UN Intergovernmental Panel on Climate Change**'s 2018 *Special Report: Global Warming of 1.5°C*: ipcc.ch/sr15.

Learn about why other countries and regions of the world apply the **Precautionary Principle** to decisions that affect communities, societies, and natural systems by reading Dr. Bernard Goldstein's article in the *American Journal of Public Health*: doi.org/10.2105/ajph.91.9.1358.

Research the right **electric bike** for your purposes. This list hits most buckets and budgets: Swagtron EB5 Pro (found at Walmart), VanMoof, Biktrix, Priority Bicycles, Niner Bikes.

Discover companies that are offering sustainable **energy solutions to corporations** and communities: 3Degrees (3degreesinc .com), BoxPower (boxpower.io), Tesla (tesla.com/powerwall), and InPipe Energy (inpipeenergy.com).

Find out the essential requirements for turning your deck, balcony, and property into a **wildlife sanctuary** from the National Wildlife Federation: nwf.org/garden-for-wildlife/certify.

Give **building materials** another life by donating or buying them used at Habitat for Humanity's ReStore locations: habitat.org/ restores.

Looking to live small or build a **tiny home** that perfectly fits your needs? Check out Artisan Tiny House: artisantinyhouse.com/ artisan-tiny-house-process.

Browse an **Amsterdam grocery store** by visiting Organic: laren amsterdam.organicfoodforyou.nl.

Get inspired and **cook with the food you've already purchased** at Cook with What You Have: cookwithwhatyouhave.com.

Find out more about **CSAS**, including those in your area, through LocalHarvest: localharvest.org/csa/.

Try some **plant-based meat alternatives**: Tofurky (tofurky.com), Beyond Meat (beyondmeat.com), and Meati (meati.com).

Instead of throwing them out, consider having your **jeans repaired** by Denham: denhamthejeanmaker.com/en/about/service-co.html.

Shop for **renewed clothing** at Eileen Fisher Renew (eileenfisher renew.com), and visit Trove (trove.co) and The Renewal Workshop (renewalworkshop.com) to find out what brands use their renewal services.

Discover companies that are creating **sustainable textiles for clothing manufacturers** from new and revalorized sources: Bolt Threads (boltthreads.com), Evrnu (evrnu.com), and Worn Again (wornagain.co.uk).

Learn about **water scarcity** through the World Wildlife Fund: worldwildlife.org/threats/water-scarcity.

The US Environmental Protection Agency website on **waste** provides information on how waste is managed in this country and how you can reduce and manage your own waste: epa.gov/environmental-topics/land-waste-and-cleanup-topics.

A growing number of companies are making it easier to manage **hard-to-recycle items**, including Ridwell (ridwell.com) and TerraCycle (terracycle.com).

Find out about **Extended Producer Responsibility** laws within the US for specific industries and how regulations in other countries affect waste streams and environmental pollution by reading journal articles on the topic: sciencedirect.com/topics/earth-and-planetary-sciences/extended-producer-responsibility.

Ecovative Design is using mycelium—mushrooms—to make **plant-based meat, packaging, and textiles**, and they'll even help you grow your own: ecovativedesign.com.

Shop for **upcycled accessories** made from excess materials otherwise destined for landfill at Looptworks: looptworks.com.

Refresh your wardrobe sustainably at Rent the Runway: renttherunway.com.

Investigate **toy rentals** at Whirli (whirli.com) and Rent That Toy! (rent-that-toy.com).

Access worksheets for charting your **sustainability action plan** on my website: kategaertner.com.

About the Author

KATE GAERTNER is a leading sustainability expert with twenty-five years of corporate and entrepreneurial experience. She is the founder and CEO of TripleWin Advisory, a consultancy that educates and supports organizations in the implementation of business circularity measures in order to conserve natural resources and promote material reuse, recycling, and product longevity. She holds a master of science in sustainable management from the University of Wisconsin, an MBA from the Wharton School, and an AB from Dartmouth College.

Kate serves on the board of the XXcelerate Fund, a business accelerator and fund for women-led businesses, and has held management positions at XM Satellite Radio, Ziff Davis Media, and Time Inc., as well as worked as a strategic consultant to Fortune 500 companies developing go-to-market business cases. She also founded a sustainable women's activewear lifestyle brand, OMALA.

Kate is married with two great kids and lives in downtown Portland, Oregon.

KATEGAERTNER.COM

Plant Sustainability Seeds in Your Life

Do you feel empowered to live more sustainably and act as an agent of sustainable change for others? Keep up your momentum with tools to guide your journey toward a life well lived. On Kate's website you'll find:

A Quiz: Determine your key value drivers and suggested sustainability measures.

Tips, Tricks, and Links: Strategies for implementing sustainability actions in your life, a sixty-card box set to keep you motivated all year long, and links to movements and organizations that are moving the dial on climate change.

Worksheets: Download worksheets, checklists, and action plans to customize and personalize your sustainability goals.

Workshops: Sixty- to ninety-minute live, interactive events that help you maintain a growth mindset, identify your passions, and target sustainability measures that are just right for you and your team. Check the online event calendar for upcoming workshops.

Program: This multi-week, guided, self-paced sustainability course walks you through the importance and value of personal sustainability. You'll learn how to categorize measures through the small, medium, large (S-M-L) sustainability bucket approach so that your efforts are doable, measurable, and meaningful. Start your sustainability journey today.

kategaertner.com
🐦 @kategaertner
📷 @katetriplewin
f kategaertner
in Kate Gaertner

Bring *Planting a Seed* to Your Organization

Build the "sustainability muscle" of your employees. Kate has a decade of proven success involving teams and organizations in advancing their corporate social responsibility initiatives. She can provide the frameworks and tools to implement sustainability measures successfully in employees' lives as well as grow the foundational knowledge of your company's loyal brand ambassadors.

Bulk Buy: Buy copies of *Planting a Seed* for your team, department, or division and receive a complimentary sixty-minute stakeholder engagement workshop. Contact Kate about bulk discounts and special offers, including custom editions that can incorporate a foreword from your CEO or company-branded cover design.

Workshops: Bring *Planting a Seed* training into your organization either virtually or in person. Kate offers stakeholder engagement workshops for employees, suppliers, and green teams. She will show you how to implement business circularity so your teams and departments can catalyze sustainable action. Options range from sixty-minute workshops to half- and full-day team-building on actionable sustainability measures to achieve impactful, carbon-reducing results.

Speaking: Kate's keynote speeches focus on how businesses can create long-term value with new purchasing and consumption models and circular business practices. Contact Kate to speak at one of your organizational events.

triplewinadvisory.com
✉ kate@triplewinadvisory.com
🐦 @triplewinadvise
📷 @triplewinadvisory
ⓕ triplewinadvisory